A Spring in my Step

Joan McDonnell

The Collins Press

Published in 2004 by
The Collins Press,
West Link Park,
Doughcloyne,
Wilton,
Cork

British Library Cataloguing in Publication data.

Printed in Ireland by ColourBooks Ltd.

This book is printed on uncoated paper manufactured with the greatest possible care for the environment.

Typesetting by The Collins Press

Typeface Palatino 10 point

ISBN: 1-903464-60-9

Cover image: Stepping Stones, © Getty Images

CONTENTS

෴

JOAN MCDONNELL left school at fifteen and worked
at numerous jobs in Limerick, eventually becoming
a lab technician with a US multi-national. In 1973 she married
the writer Vincent McDonnell after a three-week romance,
and moved to London. In 1984 they returned to Ireland
with their young son. She now lives in County Cork
where she manages a medical centre.

*To Vincent my husband,
and my son Vincent, with love always*

FOREWORD

❦

Joan McDonnell spoke to me on the Gay Byrne Show one day in 1988 about the publication of her husband Vince's book and we were able to give her some help. I knew nothing about her at the time, and she never mentioned that she was handicapped. Vince wasn't the only writer in their house. A few years later, I happened to use an expression on the show which is a standard, well-worn showbiz put down, to describe, say, a comedian, who is supposed to be funny and isn't – '... he's about as funny as polio'.

Joan picked up on the phrase and wrote me a letter which I read out on air. It got a great reaction from our listeners, so much so that, with some amendments, it forms the opening chapter of this book. Here was a young woman, a polio sufferer, who was saying that polio doesn't always have to be unfunny. Not for her, anyway.

We all tend to be reticent, or awkward, or ill at ease in the face of disability. Most assuredly, we go out of our way to try not to offend, and it is a very strictly observed taboo in showbusiness that you do not make fun of handicap in any way. Whatever else you try to get a laugh from, not that. You do not mock the afflicted.

Whenever I see someone who is severely handicapped, obviously from birth, I wonder at what precise moment in their young life did the realisation come that they were different from everyone else and – worse – that it would always be so. And how did they react? And how did they cope? And who did they talk to about it? And in the still small hours of the night, what was in their thoughts?

And it is with a sense of relief and iuplif that we read Joan's version of what it's like to be stricken with polio – the fun she's had as a result of it and the hilarious attempts she made to overcome it. Consider this exchange, after she put a lump of timber in her shoe to disguise her limp and show everyone that she could walk as straight as anybody else:

'Notice anything?' I ask.
They look hard. 'Yeah, you're walking funny,' they say.
'No I'm not, I'm walking straight.'
'So you are. It just looks funny, you walking straight.'

Talk about a slight undermining of confidence! Anyone else getting a verbal belt like that would have been in therapy for nine years, but not our Joan. She just picks herself up, dusts herself off and starts all over again. And as for attracting boyfriends: any pretty girl can garner a bevy of admirers, disguising their acne and panting with uncertain lust. But a girl with a misshapen leg and a bad limp has a rather more difficult time. That is the reality Joan has to cope with, and it did not deter her one iota. Her description of her efforts in that regard are simply hilarious.

She has a great story to tell, but then, a lot of people have that. It's not enough. You have to be able to tell it. And in my opinion, Joan tells her story with verve and wit and insight and some very fine writing. And totally devoid of any suggestion of victim-hood.

I hesitate to use words such as 'inspiring' and 'indomitable spirit', although they both come to mind, so I'll just say that the book is a splendid achievement, and if in any way we sparked the process all those years ago on radio, we are happy to take a bow on that account.

GAY BYRNE
December 2003

1

THE JOURNEY

❦

I am eight years old and, officially declared to be handicapped, I am about to undertake the greatest adventure of my young life. I am going on a long train journey all by myself. As I stand on the platform at Colbert Station in Limerick this sunny summer's morning in 1959, I can hardly believe that when I return this evening I will not be handicapped any longer, but just another little girl, like all my friends.

I will have two good legs like all little girls should possess. The thin, deformed and shortened left limb will have disappeared and been replaced by a brand new one. My only concern is whether Our Lady, who lives in Knock in County Mayo and who is going to perform this miracle, will have an exact match for my good right leg.

I'm a little confused as to exactly how the miracle will be achieved. Will my hated, withered leg fall off and a new one grow in its place? If this is so, will I then have to wait weeks for the new one to grow to its correct length? And what if it doesn't grow long enough, or just keeps on growing and growing?

Even to my eight-year-old intelligence, this seems an unlikely way of replacing deformed limbs. What's more likely is that they will have a supply of replacement limbs at Knock and I will be able to choose one for myself. Then it's off with the old one and on with the new. It will simply be like one of the many operations I've already had, only this time there will be no horrid scar visible to mark the join. I know Our Lady would never stand for that. And as well as that, I'd been shown a picture of someone who had got a new nose in a miracle at Knock and they had no scars on their face.

As I stand on the platform in my red coat, with a blue cross pinned on its front, I feel like the most important person in the world. I have no envy for the little girl in the blue dress with her parents, seeing off someone on a stretcher. She wears black patent sandals with silver buckles, and her legs above the white ankle socks are smooth and straight and equal in length. But she isn't going to Knock.

My two legs will be exactly like hers when I return. No longer will I have to wear my heavy, black boots, nor the calliper that's attached to the left one. I too will be able to wear white ankle socks and patent black sandals with silver buckles. I'll be able to run and play like all the other children on our street without fear of falling. I won't be called Hopalong Cassidy, or cripple, or hand-icapped, or 'that one with the lame leg' any more.

The station is crowded with people and I hold on tight to my father's hand, a little frightened of the crush. There are invalids in wheelchairs and on stretchers, and others with crutches. Men and women in uniforms scurry about, helping people onto the train. There are some who appear to have two good legs and hands and proper noses too, but they also wear blue crosses. I wonder what sort of miracle they are expecting.

I can hardly wait to get on the train. If I could support my weight on my left leg, I would be hopping impatiently from one leg to the other. But I have to stand with most of my weight on my right leg, and even after a short while I begin to tire.

The people in the wheelchairs and the stretchers are loaded on first. At last it is my turn. A steward takes me from my father and helps me up onto the train. 'Bye, love,' my father says, using his regular term of endearment whenever we part. In my eight years there have been many such partings. But this I know will be the final one. I will not have to go away to hospital any more for further operations on my leg. It will be an end to that – to the parting and the loneliness and the pain.

Once on the train, a woman takes my hand and leads me to my seat. It's by the window and I look out but there is no sign of my father. Panic grips me and I am about to cry out that I don't want to go when he appears outside the window. He smiles and winks at me, and I relax. I know then that I have to go to Knock. There are so many people depending on my going and being cured. I know my father wants me to have a new leg and I can't let him down.

Whistles sound and doors slam. Then the train jerks and jerks again and the station begins to move. It is the most amazing sight I have ever seen. There I am sitting in my seat while the buildings and people are moving past me. By the time I've recovered from the shock, my father has slipped by and is lost to sight.

The buildings gather speed and the moving rails outside the window become a blur. While our train stands still, my father and the railway station and all those other people are heading for Knock! No wonder the train is frantically blowing its whistle. It's being left behind.

It takes a little while for me to realise that in fact we are moving. Once I realise this, I relax and begin to enjoy the experience. The train picks up speed and begins to sway gently. Outside it goes clickety-clack, clickety-clack and I think that must be its song.

The world outside the window now becomes a blur. The dark shapes of trees and poles whiz by at enormous speed. But in the distance, now that we've left the city behind, I can see houses and green fields and cows grazing. A man in a field raises his hand and waves to me. I am tempted to wave back but I'm much too shy.

But I'm not too shy to enjoy my sense of freedom. I am eight years old and going, all on my own, on a journey of nearly 100 miles. It is a very thrilling adventure for someone who is handicapped, who has polio and a bad leg and is on the way to Knock, in County Mayo, to be cured.

No one has ever told me what polio (I always pronounced it polo) is and so I once asked my father about it. He was the man to ask because he claimed to know everything about everything.

'Polo?' he'd asked, looking at me in a most peculiar way. 'It's a game played with sticks and a ball by men on horseback. It's a bit like hurling without horses, love.'

I knew what hurling was all right. Sometimes the boys in the street played it with sticks and a tin can. They were always very rough and wild when they played and it was best to keep out of their way. The game usually ended with black eyes and bleeding noses and women with big bellies waddling from their houses to rescue Tommy or Johnny or Paddy before he ended up black and blue all over.

Now my father's answer not only cleared up the question of what polo was, but also explained why I was handicapped like Lester Piggott. He rode horses and I knew that he too was often handicapped. But what did handicap mean? This, I decided, was another question for the oracle.

'It's got to do with putting weights in a horse's saddlebags,' my father told me. His look now was even more peculiar.

But it was all making perfect sense to me. I realised that I must have been one of those weights and had fallen out of the saddlebag. Now I needed to know where this had happened. But when I asked the oracle if I had fallen out of Lester Piggott's saddlebag during the Grand National, he gave me an exasperated look, and began to mutter that it was well past time for 'Ha Bu'. At that point I decided it was time to make myself scarce.

So with this last question still unanswered, I'm now on my way to Knock and a miracle cure. What with having polio and being handicapped and with a bad leg as well, I know I'll require a big one. And as the train is crowded with invalids, most of them worse than me, I realise for the first time that there is an awful lot of handicap and polio about.

The blue paper cross, with my name on it, pinned to my coat, declares to the world that I am an invalid. Now, even at eight, I detest that word, which I pronounce in valid, and which I've learned at school means not acceptable. But there's nothing wrong with me to make me unacceptable. I am fit and strong and ready for anything. I wouldn't even know that I have a limp except that people keep telling me I have. They sometimes go so far as to demonstrate how well I limp. In fact most of them limp better than I do. But they aren't going to Knock.

I had been so excited as the train pulled out of the station, what with looking forward to the journey and the promised miracle at the end of it; and knowing too that I was the envy of all the family, this added spice to my pleasure. But the pleasure is short-lived when everyone starts saying the rosary. This worries me because I think I might be cured before we even reach Knock and will be put off the train. It takes three rosaries altogether to reach Claremorris where, to my relief, I find I still have the polio, the bad leg and the limp.

Here we are put on buses that take us onto Knock. When we arrive there are stewards waiting to help us off the bus. One of them lifts me down and puts me in a wheelchair. 'I can walk,' I say rather indignantly.

'You can't walk here,' he says, tucking a blanket firmly about me, and handing me into the care of a nurse. I would have asked her if I could walk – after my confinement on the train and bus I want to run – but I'm much too shy.

I am now beginning to worry about Knock. I've been brought here for a miracle cure and yet within minutes of arriving find myself in a wheelchair. It's just as well my mother or father can't see me.

So I'm off with Florence Nightingale, attracting, in my opinion, undeserved sympathetic looks wherever we go. I'm aware that the longer I spend in the wheelchair the harder it will be to get out.

I attend Mass in the wheelchair and later, as I'm wheeled about the grounds, have what seems like gallons of Holy Water sprinkled on me by elderly women. One lifts up the rug, much to my consternation, and sloshes another gallon on my legs. At the same time she's praying aloud for me to be cured. I'm sorely tempted to leap out of the chair, but I know if I do so, she'll drop dead from fright. It really is a quandary. Here I am at Knock, expecting a cure for my polio and all the rest, and it seems as if it will require a miracle just to get out of the wheelchair.

The day passes and I wonder when my miracle is to take place. So far, no one seems to have been cured. I ask Florence about my miracle and she smiles sadly and pats me on the head. She looks so sad that I decide not to ask her again.

Perhaps Our Lady is away in Lourdes, I think, and I've been sent here on the wrong day. Or perhaps they've run out of left legs and are awaiting a new delivery. Whatever the reason, it doesn't bother me any more. The only thing worrying me now is the fear that they might give me this wheelchair instead.

By late afternoon nature takes its course. I need to go to the toilet and my Florence wheels me there. Now my eight-year-old sense of decency, coupled with the fact that there is no one here to frighten to death, takes over from my shyness. When Florence takes my arm and says, 'I'll help you in,' I think to myself, 'Not likely!'

I'm up and out of the chair in a flash while Florence stands there astonished. 'My God, you can walk,' she exclaims. Walk! I could run if it wasn't for the fact that I'm crippled from being confined in the damn chair.

I have a great day in Knock, despite my polio not being cured and not getting the promised new leg. But after spending so much time in the wheelchair I realise it wouldn't have been fair to cure me when there are so many others who can't walk at all. That's what I have learned this day. And that is to be my miracle – that knowledge that I don't need a miracle after all.

2

THE BIG LADY

❦

My arrival into the world on 19 July 1951 is greeted with both excitement and panic. The excitement is for the new arrival, despite the fact that it is a hard struggle to rear the three other children already in the family. The panic, on the other hand, is caused by the umbilical cord being wound about my neck.

Unlike most babies, I emerge into the world from under the proverbial head of cabbage, not screaming but gasping, and with only the midwife between me and a quick exit. She is the woman for a crisis, and with an exclamation of Jesus, Mary and St Joseph, she throws herself on her knees before a large picture of the Sacred Heart and starts to entreat every saint in heaven to help her.

My mother is made of sterner stuff. And though she knows that St Jude is the man to turn to in hopeless cases, she is also well aware that he is unlikely to have had much experience of childbirth. There isn't much that he, or indeed any of the saints can do right now. 'Will you get up off your knees you *amadán*,' she berates the stricken midwife, 'and for the love of God do something for the child!'

Whether it's my mother's scathing words or the love of God bit that does the trick will never be known. But one or both of them work, for the midwife, with alacrity, obeys the command. She rises quickly from her knees and somehow unwinds the cord whilst at the same time still imploring the help of God and all his saints.

Able to get a breath at last, I manage a weak cry or two. And then, getting the hang of it, I bawl stridently. At this, the midwife throws herself on her knees again to offer up her thanks and my mother lets her be, enjoining her own prayers of thanks, with those of the distraught saviour.

I weigh 6lb 12ozs, and I'm known, for a time at least, as The Big Lady. So it must be quite a substantial cabbage I was found under. But as they already know in heaven that three other children have been sent down in baskets to our house, they are no doubt also aware that food is always in great demand. God, or more than likely Our Lady, for surely she's the one who would do the cooking up there, must have realised that a large head of cabbage won't go amiss.

With such a perilous beginning to my life, surely things can only get better from now on. But it seems as if they want me back in heaven, and when the first attempt fails, are only too willing to try again. So, though I'm a quiet baby, a good feeder (presumably not on the cabbage) and I sleep and thrive, tipping the scales at fifteen pounds by four months, a threat to my continued well being is already in motion.

When my father carries me in his arms to the City Home Hospital, just a stone's throw up the road from where we live, the doctors there diagnose this threat – high temperature with a rash – as scarlet fever. They shake their heads and pronounce the prognosis as not good.

As a consequence of this my mother goes hurrying home to Killeely for the Holy Water, miraculous intervention being the only answer in a time of crisis (with the exception of an unfortunate midwife faced with a baby in the process of being strangled by an umbilical cord in the dead of night).

When my mother returns with the Holy Water I have been placed in isolation and she is not allowed to have any contact with me. She is told she can look at me through a window, but as the window is high up on the wall and my mother is of low stature, she has to make do with standing on an orange box (they must keep it at the hospital for use by people such as her) and peeping through the glass at me. A kind nurse takes care of the Holy Water and sprinkles some on me whenever she has the opportunity.

Each day my mother makes the relatively short journey on foot from home to the hospital, on occasions reluctantly accompanied by my grumbling father, who complains that visiting sick babies is a woman's job and beneath his dignity. But as he too is of low stature, like my mother, and has to make use of the orange box as well, it is probably this affront to his manly dignity that bothers him.

I can only imagine how upsetting it must be for my parents, seeing their tiny baby all but lost in a large cot, undoubtedly showing signs of sickness and distress, and restrained from moving about by some sort of harness. My mother's natural instinct is surely to rush in, pick me up and comfort me. But she is as much restrained by the rules and regulations as I am by the harness.

She is much more worried by that harness than by the scarlet fever. Despite the rules and regulations and good old-fashioned fear of authority, she voices her concern about the dangers of the harness, only to be told that it is hospital policy. She should thank God her child is getting such good treatment, she is told, especially when there are those more worthy (though obviously not as sick) who have to make do with private nursing at home and a twice-daily visit from their doctor.

Aware that she isn't going to change anything, she decides to keep quiet, and instead places her faith in the Holy Water to keep the straps well away from my neck. (Later it is rumoured that a child has been strangled in an Irish hospital with some sort of similar restraint, thus amply justifying my mother's fears, if the rumours are true.)

With the Holy Water preventing me from being strangled and, along with the medicine, fighting the scarlet fever, I can't help but get well. In a matter of weeks I am able to return home, again carried by my father in his arms because they can't afford to hire a taxi, there is no bus service and one has to be dying, or influential, to qualify for an ambulance.

Heaven again has been thwarted in its attempt to have me back, but it will bide its time and soon will make a more determined effort. Yet for the present I am safe, though still weak. I have lost a great deal of weight and am no longer worthy of the name The Big Lady.

***

Number Fourteen Hennessy Avenue, Killeely, is where we live, but to my mother it has never been home. There had been some mix up when the house was allocated to them on their return from Coventry, where they first met and were married. My mother had picked another house on the street and bitterly resented not getting it.

She is a small woman, very blunt and outspoken, from Kilmeedy in County Limerick. She is fiercely proud of her birthplace, her family and the people of that area. She detests Limerick city. She has never seen anything else here but poverty and deprivation and sickness. She rears her family as best she can, scraping by from week to week, proud that she has never had the electricity disconnected in her home because she couldn't pay the bills. She has managed this feat by using a single light bulb. All the other bulbs have been removed at her insistence by my father.

His people originally come from Tipperary and there is supposed to be some scandal in the family. An ancestor of his, perhaps his grandfather, married beneath him and was ostracised by his well-to-do family. This ancestor came to Limerick with his unsuitable bride and set up home in Vize's Field, one of Limerick's most notorious slums. Later, the family move to The Island Field, one of the first County Council Housing Schemes to take the people out of the slums and the lanes of Limerick.

My father is a small man and, with his dark hat and laughing face, is often mistaken for James Cagney. He had been married before he met my mother and has one son by his first wife. When she died shortly after their son Tom's birth, he left the boy with his grandmother and set off for England. Here he was to meet my mother and marry her.

They had some future in Coventry where they had a home and work, but for some reason, unknown even to themselves, they returned to Limerick, where they have no work and no hope, and as far as my mother is concerned, no home.

But I am happily unaware of all this and to me Number Fourteen, Hennessey Avenue is home. So, spared yet again, I return to the dampness and the poverty. I continue eating and sleeping until soon, I am sitting up and studying the world around me.

Then I begin to crawl and by 1952 I am quickly finding my feet. But following a bout of measles I keep losing them. Each time I manage to stand up, I fall down again. Something is wrong. I am taken to the City Home Hospital again but they obviously don't know very much there about falling down, for they eventually decide to send me to Dublin, where apparently they know everything.

But how am I to get to Dublin? We are too poor to even own a bicycle. Only the super rich own cars and obviously we don't count any of them amongst our friends. There is the ambulance, of course, but it only travels short distances. So there is no way of getting me to Dublin. Maybe I'm expected to walk there, but isn't that the very reason I'm being sent in the first place, for it's only in Dublin, it seems, that Limerick people can be taught how to walk properly without falling down?

My mother is naturally upset about this, and is in a very grumpy mood when she meets local politician, Steve Coughlan, in the city. 'I'll never vote for none of ye again,' she tells the bemused man in her blunt way.

'Sure what's wrong with you, Mrs Ryan?' he asks

'I have a young child due to go to Dublin,' she tells him, 'and there's no way of getting her there. The ambulance won't take her

11

and I can't afford the train.'

'Don't worry about a thing,' he says. 'I'll sort it all out for you'.

And he does. At six the following morning the ambulance calls to the house to take me to Dublin. And Steve Coughlan's kindness extends even further, as he offers to take my mother to visit me whenever he is going up to Dublin. But as she would have to stay until he is returning, or find her own way home, she cannot avail of his offer. Only once will she visit me in three years.

It doesn't take them too long in Dublin to find out that polio has paralysed my left leg. They are brilliant at the diagnosis bit, but fixing it – well, that is a different matter entirely. It is going to be a long haul – three years and three operations to be exact. I don't know what is the purpose of the operations, only that they hurt and leave horrible scars on my leg.

My parents pay me that single visit during this time. Apparently my father is away working in England and is coming home and he makes an arrangement for my mother to meet him in Dublin.

Steve Coughlan takes my mother to Dublin but she does not have much money and what she has must be spared. She feels she cannot afford to stay in lodgings in the city. So she sits all night in the railway station waiting room until my father's boat train arrives in from Dun Laoghaire at dawn the next morning.

What a sight greets them at the hospital. I am still a small baby, isolated and with my leg attached to the ceiling by wires and pulleys. I'm clearly still not going anywhere, despite all the operations.

My mother brings me a doll and the visit is very upsetting for them. When they leave to go home to Limerick, they do not know when they will see me again. But the hospital assures them they will shortly allow me the odd weekend at home, just so the family will not completely forget who I am. Yet I have already forgotten who they are. I'm a stranger now.

3

HOME AND AWAY

❧

When I return home for my first visit, the problem facing my mother is what to do with me. Because I can't walk unaided, I spend all my waking time lying on the kitchen floor or lying in my cot. This won't do, for what happens if the other children stand on me, something that is very likely when two of them are boisterous boys?

I couldn't return to Dublin with a broken right leg as well as a paralysed left one. They'd never be able to put that right and I'd probably end up staying there forever. So in order to avoid this possibility, my mother invents the play-pen, only she doesn't realise her stroke of genius at the time. She obtains a tea chest from a local shop and puts me in it. I can grab hold of the edge, pull myself up and stumble around. This I do all day, walking for what seems miles in this manner.

My visit home happens to coincide with the birth of my sister. But she will not be born at home, not after the fright I gave my mother. As she leaves the house on her way to the maternity hospital, she looks back sorrowfully at me in my tea chest and thinks to herself: 'That's the end of the attention for you.'

My sister Celia is born at the end of October 1952. My mother does not have tuppence for the bus and walks the two and a half miles to Killeely in the pouring rain, with her new baby in her arms. But this is not an unusual sight, for many of the people living in

Killeely are poor like ourselves; and the poorer they are, the more children they seem to have. Women are hardly ever seen without a prominent belly and another baby in their arms.

It is going to be difficult for my mother coping with this new baby and looking after me at the same time. Even the simple chore of washing nappies poses its own problems – water has to be heated and some sort of detergent provided – and money to buy food, never mind coal and detergent, is always in very short supply.

Drying the nappies is even more of a problem in the short, cold, sunless November days. She somehow manages to get most of the moisture out of them and then places them inside her own clothes to air them. Plastic pants, even if they were available, are a luxury she can't afford and there is no oil sheet on the cot. This means that the cot sheet, made from a flour bag, as well as the baby's clothes, can and do become soaking wet. It is a hard time for women who have small children.

So in many ways it must be a blessing to her that I am returning to Dublin and will only come home in the next three years for the odd short visit. I am one less in the house to feed and look after and she knows I will be well cared for in Dublin. I will be clean and warm and fed. I have polio, but they will be able to put that right and I will be a normal little girl again.

Operations on my leg, therapy and occasional visits home from the orthopaedic hospital in Clontarf mark the passing of the next three years. My brother Mikey is born but I have no memory of him as a baby.

Eventually, they conclude that they have done all they can for me in Clontarf, or else they've become fed up with me, for they decide to send me home for good. I am walking well enough by now with the aid of iron callipers and this seems to be as normal as I will ever get. The only thing that can help me now is a miracle and that too will be tried in its own good time.

So, with my babyhood robbed from me, I'm discharged from the hospital and return home to Limerick a toddler of a different calliper – an iron one, to be precise. It looks awful but in fact it's great. It never fails to fascinate me. There are holes in each side of the boot and the long black iron rods are inserted into those. A leather strap is then fastened around my knee and the slightest movement lifts my leg up. It's like pure magic. I love it.

My brothers and sisters are in bed when I arrive home and my father takes me upstairs to see them. There are four of them in one room – the baby, Mikey, still sleeps in my parents' bedroom. The four here share two beds, and without any form of lighting, it is dark in the room. I can make out pale blurred faces staring at me above heaped up bedclothes – a few blankets supplemented with overcoats.

They all scramble out of the beds and crowd around to have a look at me. They have seen me before, but this is different. Now they know that I am going to be staying here for good. This makes a difference to their attitude to me and mine to them.

I am equally fascinated by these kids crowding about me. I stand in the centre of them, not knowing what to do or say. My father asks me if I want to go downstairs. I want to go and I want to stay. I don't want to leave these strangers, who are my brothers and sisters, but I don't feel comfortable amongst them.

As my eyes become accustomed to the dark I notice that they seem dirty and that their nightclothes are raggy. I stand beside them clean and spruce in my blue dress and my matching furry coat that looks like a sheep has had his fleece permed and dyed. Any right-thinking sheep would have quickly disowned it.

But all this will quickly change. Soon I will be as dirty and unkempt as them. I will become used to them but they will never get used to me or come to accept me. I'm the stranger who has come among them and takes all the attention.

***

This is a whole new world for me and one that I will have to come to terms with. My father is unemployed and that is an advantage for me. Because he has so much time on his hands, he spends a great deal of it out walking. As I can now walk, even if not too well, and I don't attend school as yet, he often takes me out with him. I always ask him where's his white coat. Most of the men I have known up to now have had white coats.

I love going out for walks. I hardly knew before this that there was a sky or so much space. In the hospital I'd become used to confinement. Now I see all the houses and the people and I realise how big the world is. I'm not the only person in existence.

I take everything in when I'm out in the world. But it's so big and I tire easily. So more often than not my father ends up carrying me for most of those walks.

I don't know any baby talk. Hospitals just don't have time for that. So one day when I've tired him out and we get home, he asks, 'Do you want to go to "Ha Bu" now?' My vivid imagination comes into play.

My face lights up at a vision of mountains and valleys from a prehistoric time. Of course, I want to go to this magical land of 'Ha Bu'. So I agree delightedly. I am rather disappointed when the mountains turn out to be the stairs and the valley my bed. But I have agreed and so to bed, as Pepys was wont to say.

But I have learned a valuable lesson. What people say is not always what they mean. Even children, and that includes my own brothers and sisters, cannot be trusted. It teaches me to be wary and that in turn leads others to dislike me. They do not like my honesty either, but the conditioning of my early years will stay with me forever. They cannot understand why I am as I am.

It's because most of my childhood has been spent in hospital that I do not behave like a normal child. At least that's my excuse for being me. Hospital is an artificial environment and one not suited to someone who by rights should be living in a cave in the Stone Age. So now that I'm living in the real world, this new lifestyle takes some getting used to.

For example, I have never heard anyone swearing before – doctors and nurses don't swear. At least I never heard them say 'you better f***ing walk or else'. But there is a great deal of swearing to be heard now. Much force can be put behind the swear words. It's all a great novelty for me. And as I need to be heard and to be the centre of attention, I am f***ing and blinding every second word. I'm delighted too to be adding new words to what is a very limited vocabulary.

But my mother soon puts a stop to this. I suppose it was amusing for a while, but there is a limit to her humour, especially when I begin to swear at her. She chastises me each time I use a swear word and so I stop – officially at least. But unofficially, on the street, I still use them. The other children are both frightened and fascinated by my behaviour. They think that thunder and lightning will come if someone swears, and they threaten me with this. I'm terrified of thunder and lightning, but I'm still willing to tempt fate. Little do I know that fate is only biding its time.

Money is scarce and TB is rife. Most people take out some form of insurance, just to cover the costs of a possible funeral. So when a man from The Friendly Insurance Company comes to the area selling what is known as the 'penny insurance', my mother decides to avail of the chance. The whole family is insured for eight pence a week. But I am not included. I am too much of a risk. Even The Friendly Insurance Company doesn't want to befriend me.

By 1956 the doctors want to take my calliper away. I don't know why, as without it I can't walk at all. But despite that, I'm being sent to the orthopaedic hospital in Croom, nine miles from Limerick, to relieve me of the calliper.

It's a strange place. They have huge cave-like structures over the beds of people who've been operated on, to keep them warm. Being a prehistoric sort of person, I'd feel perfectly at home in them – except that Thomas Edison must have broken his leg at some stage and fitted these cavern-like structures with dozens of electric light bulbs, to pass away the time. He should have stuck to the gramophone!

I don't like it in Croom. They do terrible things to me here, supposedly for my own good. One day I'm placed on a trolley, a plastic cap is put on my head and I'm wheeled away. I don't know where I'm going, but it takes four people to wheel the trolley with just me on it. I feel really proud. Joey, the driver, makes me laugh as he wheels me into an operating theatre, but I don't know that's what it is. There's no such thing as pre-med so I get to have a good look at all the weird and dangerous looking equipment.

There are great big silver drums with steam coming out of them. I don't know if they are going to put me into one of them! I'm lifted off the trolley and onto the operating table. Above my head there is a large disc. Judging by the number of light bulbs in it, Edison has been here too.

It's not my first time in an operating theatre but I don't remember the other occasions. Now I'm awed and quiet and not a little apprehensive as I contemplate my fate. Joey calls my name and I look back at him. At that very same moment I feel a sharp prick on my arm. There it is a cheap – mean trick. Joey has tricked me and a nurse has pricked me. Another fine example of the behaviour of sneaky hospital staff. I don't like Joey any more, but before I can really work on it, I'm out for the count.

Some time later I'm woken by someone slapping my face really hard. Some sadistic Florence Nightingale is really giving me the once over, and I've done nothing wrong. I have just had an operation and I'm getting some TLC, hospital-style. I throw up.

When I eventually wake up properly, I'm aware that my leg feels very heavy. It's in plaster. The plaster's so heavy that I'm certain I won't be able to lift my leg ever again.

A cage has been placed over my feet in case they run away. I'm told it's to keep the weight of the blankets off my leg, but after being beaten up, how can I believe anything I'm told? My feet feel very cold under that cage, in contrast to my face which is hot from the blows I've been dealt, and I wonder if Florence has beaten the wrong end.

Time passes slowly and I'm confined to bed. All I have to do is wiggle my toes for the doctors. That seems to really please them. Odd people, doctors. The plaster is on my leg all this time and the itch is unbearable. It's so bad I feel like bashing my leg against any hard surface and smashing the hated plaster to smithereens.

Indeed, if one could never move their leg, the itch would surely make them discover some way of moving it. Maybe that's how orthopaedic hospitals get people walking again. It's got nothing to do with medical skill – just drop a little itching powder down inside a plaster of paris and anyone will move.

The days pass in this same dreary way. The plaster remains and so does the itch. But the nurses are kind and friendly and I'm not beaten up again. Yet I yearn to clamber from the bed and run around, to go out into the world I glimpse through the window. I want to be home again in Killeely, to play on the street with the other children and to go walking with my father.

I miss him, just as I miss my mother and home. The bed here is soft and the sheets are clean and smooth and there are no piles of overcoats to weigh me down. But I still wish I were back in my own cot at home, even though it's much too small to accommodate me. I could never share the bed with my sisters because they might break my leg, which is hardly thicker than my wrist. However, a broken leg would be much more preferable than what I endure now.

No one has been to visit me and I envy the other patients their visitors. Sometimes I wonder if I will ever return home, and at night I often lie awake and think that I will never see any of my family again. No one tells me how long I will be here, if the plaster will ever be removed, or if I will be able to walk again when it is. I try not to cry but sometimes in the darkness the tears flow freely. There is no one to hear and no one to come and cheer me with any comforting words.

***

Christmas comes and so does Santa. He brings me a doll. He sits on my bed and his beard speaks to me. I keep staring at it as it moves up and down. He seems to have been badly assembled and I feel that he's going to fall apart. I hope he won't fall apart on my bed.

He is very thin for a Santa Claus, which doesn't seem right. Maybe hospitals don't leave out food like other children do. I keep staring at his moving beard and then I scream and scream. I feel that might shift him before he does come apart. I know it's Christmas but Santa can go and frighten someone else, preferably the Nightingale.

The new year of 1957 dawns and I'm still in the hospital. The nurses seem to have carried over their policy of not beating up the patients any more to the new year, so I can relax and take an interest in what is going on around me.

Every now and again a person appears in the ward with a battered green box. They take this to the bed of a patient, which is then screened off. From behind the screens there comes a loud whirring noise. I assume this comes from whatever is in that green box and not from the patient. How I long to know what it is, but no one will tell me. It's a state secret.

One day, the green box again arrives in the ward. This time it's brought to my bed. At last my curiosity will be satisfied. The screens are pulled around my bed and the box is opened. To my horror, it contains a Black & Decker Chain Saw. No wonder the contents are a state secret! I wonder what they are going to do with the saw – probably chop me up into little bits and reassemble me. I know now why Santa had been about to fall apart.

I'm lying on my back on the bed and a pillow is now placed over my face. No one explains anything. I have been brought here to Croom, supposedly to be cured – I'm not sure of what – and now they are going to cut my leg off just because I've complained about the itch. Only I don't know why they want to smother me as well. Maybe they're frightened that I'll shout for help.

I hear the roar of the saw and feel a breeze. Then I sense a huge weight being lifted off my leg. I try to peep out from beneath the pillow but it's pressed even firmer against my face. Now I feel little pricks along my leg every now and again and then I'm finally released. They must realise that I won't shout for help, even under torture, and have decided to let me be.

From their reaction, I think I'm supposed to be surprised and delighted to see my leg after all those months. But I'm not. It's horrible. It's red and purple and the skin is peeling. It seems even thinner than before. It has pined away in that plaster. A nurse now gently carries me to the bathroom and lowers me into a bath of lovely warm water. Here she washes off most of the old skin. 'There you are,' she says cheerfully. 'All good as new.'

'Oh yeah,' I think, 'pull the other one.' On second thoughts though, better not. I might fall and end up here for good.

Over the coming days I find out that whatever they've done here doesn't appear to have worked. I still have to wear the calliper. But what do I care when I can scratch again. That, after all, is sheer bliss. And though my left leg is woefully thin and much shorter than my right one, the doctors seem delighted.

***

So I am discharged shortly afterwards into the great big world beyond the window that I had watched with such yearning. I leave the hospital, goose-stepping like Hitler, at least with my left leg. The nurses are a little sad to see me go and indeed I feel a little sad myself as I venture out into the world. It's to be a new world – one that I have not as yet experienced – but one where I will have to quickly learn to survive or perish.

4

LEARNING THE LESSONS

❦

My first lesson in survival in the world is when I go to school for the first time. I start there soon after being discharged from Croom, attending what was known then as the 'babies' school. When I learn of the name I feel that I should have gone there years before. I imagine hundreds of babies in smelly nappies, bawling their heads off. But I soon discover that these are no babies – they are five-year-old hooligans. And I'd foolishly thought that hospitals were violent places. I know I'll have to grow up quickly if I am to survive now in school.

My first day at school dawns. My mother gets me ready and, apart from the usual washing and dressing, there is the extra task of strapping the calliper to my leg. Finally, I am ready to take my first steps into the great big world. Accompanied by my sister Celia we head off for the school. It is not very far, yet I travel there in a battered go-car because I can only walk very slowly. It would take me forever to get there if I had to half goose-step all the way.

I am apprehensive as I enter the school building, with so many children running about and laughing and making a great deal of noise. My mother approaches the headmistress and explains about my situation. Then she leaves me. The teacher takes me by the hand and leads me into the classroom. I'm terrified at the thought of being left all on my own but Celia stays back to be with me in my class.

Despite her presence, I am still very timid and frightened and I shrink into my shell. The other children sense this and, like all children, they are streaked with cruelty. Celia senses the situation and, ashamed of me, leaves me alone.

At break time I stand stiffly against the wall just outside the door that leads to the playground, terrified that a child will bump into me and I will fall. I'm not afraid of getting hurt; that isn't the problem. It's the embarrassment I will have to endure if I fall that inhibits me – that and trying to get back up, not an easy thing to do while wearing those horrible irons.

Each child that passes in and out of the school can see that I am different – for one thing, I have ugly irons on my leg – and feel it their right to slap me hard across the face. Each slap brings the tears closer and closer but not once do I raise my hand to my face to ease the pain or to protect myself. I bite my lip and fight back the tears. I do not think of retaliating because I know that any one of them would make mincemeat out of me. I wonder where Celia is, she who is supposed to protect me.

The bell goes. It's a relief to return to the classroom. Here I discover that I love learning. I want to learn everything. We sing the alphabet:

Abcdefg, hijklmnop,
Lmnop, qrst, uvw, xyz.
Xyz, sugar on your bread
When you have it eaten,
Jump into bed.

It is wonderful, and I will never forget it. But my pleasure at learning the alphabet and numbers is somewhat spoiled by the knowledge that I will have to face the playground again.

Our break time is known as *sos*, but I feel that it would be more aptly depicted by the letters SOS. I am to live in constant dread of it. But after some weeks, hope and salvation beckons. During break, many of the new children run from the school yard and head for home. Gathering all my courage one day, I decide to seek salvation and run with the posse.

Any teacher worth her salt should catch me. But they don't. Because I'm only capable of hobbling along and as I appear easy to catch, they ignore me and go full pelt after the quicker children. As they herd them back to the school, still having to dash after the odd one who makes a break for freedom, I'm left alone.

Perhaps each teacher left me to someone else, but whatever the reason, I suddenly find I have the street to myself. I'm free at last and feel exhilarated. I have escaped from the school and will never have to return there again. It has been so easy that I want to run and jump and skip with joy. I cannot do so but that doesn't dampen my happiness.

It takes my mother to do that. As soon as I get home, she takes me by the hand and marches me back again. There is no go-car this time and I have to stumble along beside her, trying to keep up. But I have learned a valuable lesson. There can be no point to running home at break time if I'm going to be marched straight back again.

I survive my first weeks and I'm now considered a veteran, well capable of going to and from the school with just my sister Celia to accompany me. There is not to be the luxury of travelling in the go-car again. But that journey to and from the school turns out to be the worst part of the day for me.

Celia is supposed to accompany me but she soon deserts me and I find myself making the journey alone. Celia is only five years of age and she bitterly resents having to be my guardian. She doesn't even want to be associated with me. After all, I'm different. I walk with a limp and that makes me less of a person in everyone's eyes. And naturally too, Celia prefers to be with her own friends.

Consequently, I find myself on my own and I am a sitting duck for anyone who wants to prove themselves a hero by showing that they are capable of beating up a defenceless child, moreover, one who is supposed to be special. But I am only special at home and then only in the eyes of my parents. Everyone else hates my special status, not least my own brothers and sisters.

I want to be like everyone else. I don't want to be special and so I try to behave like all the other children. I try to run as they do, but as my left leg tends to stray in front of my right, very often I fall.

One day on my way home from school it happens – one of the most frightening experiences of my young life so far. I'm running as best I can and a little boy is running beside me. Inevitably though, I fall over and I bring down the little boy as well. He screams, but I do not cry. I'm learning to be tough and as I am falling down all the time, I'm used to getting hurt and have learned not to cry.

Now, as I pick myself up from the ground, I'm grabbed very roughly and pushed up against a garden fence. My assailant is a girl of about seventeen and she begins to slap my face over and over again. My breath goes. I find myself in a state of shock. Then I scream and scream – the first time I have cried out loud. But there is no respite. It is only when two women across the street shout at the girl, that she stops and lets me go.

By now I am crying hysterically and I try to stop before I get home. But I am still sobbing when I get in and when my mother asks me what happened I become hysterical again, something I have rarely done. She eventually gets out of me what has happened and I have never seen her so angry. She goes off and confronts my assailant and gives her a piece of her mind. I want her to beat her to a pulp and I begin to get a glimmer of what it is to be wronged and to want vengeance.

The incident teaches me a valuable lesson. I am different and will always be different, and will always be an easy target for the bully. So I have to make a choice. I will have to keep on being such a target and become a cry baby from being beaten up all the time or I will have to become a loner.

So at the ripe old age of six, I make the decision that I will keep to myself. If I am to survive my childhood in one piece, then I know that I have to avoid other children going to and from school. And so I learn the art of survival. School becomes a place for learning, nothing more. I become a model pupil and keep to myself in the playground, refusing to mix with other children.

The only place where I can now play without fear of assault is in my own territory, with our neighbours' children. So whatever fun I miss at school, I more than make up for at home. On my own territory I am a different person, one that my classmates would not recognise.

The street is our playground. Anything there is like a magnet to us. So when a horse cart – minus the horse – is left there, we immediately surround it. It isn't that unusual to see a cart without a horse in our area. Often men actually pull the cart because they cannot afford a horse.

Now all the children are climbing up on to the cart and sliding down. It looks like great fun. I try and try to get up on the cart, but the other children keep getting up before me. In the end, in sheer frustration, I swear at them. They stop their play and stare at me in amazement.

'Now thunder and lightning will come,' they threaten, trying to frighten me.

'I don't care,' I say. But I do, especially when I see big drops of rain begin to fall, a sure sign of thunder on the way. Moments later lightning flashes across the sky and is followed immediately by the rumble of thunder. I run into the house and hide under the stairs, convinced that I have caused this to happen. That's it, I decide. No more swearing. I'm cured forever.

The more of a loner I become, the more my imagination comes into play. My imagination is very fertile and I take everything literally. I constantly live in fear of many threats. When it comes to punishment at home, I am not treated differently to the others. I am punished like all the rest.

During this time, I don't lose contact with the hospital, for I have to have a check-up every few months to see if I am still limping properly. I have no problems with limping, though. The problem is trying to get to the hospital for the check-up. It is miles from where we live and there is no direct bus route. It's enough to make one a bus hijacker.

An ambulance is the ideal means of transport to get me to and from the hospital, but ambulances don't seem to want to take people who find it difficult to walk. In a perfect *Catch-22* situation, if I could walk, I could travel in the ambulance; but being as I find it difficult to walk, I can't go in the ambulance.

After one check-up, at which I've been deemed to be limping properly, and also given good news in that I can soon dispense with the callipers, if not the horrible black boots that go with them, we are leaving the hospital when my mother sees an ambulance going to Limerick. But they won't take us, despite the fact that I am limping properly, because we aren't Hungarian refugees. My mother is furious and returns to the hospital and berates them. 'What kind of a country is this that we have to be Hungarian to get a lift in an ambulance?' she demands. I don't know exactly what happens – maybe they make us honorary Hungarians for the day – because we do eventually get the lift.

I am learning to live with myself, to survive and I'm no longer really aware that I have a problem with my leg. I am able to do the things that other children do, even if in my own way and in my own time. I am no longer unhappy because of 'the sore leg' which is how it is most often referred to. But that is about to change.

The reality of my situation really only hits me for the first time when I am about to receive my First Holy Communion. It's the biggest day in the life of any little girl and she has her dreams of what she will look like on this special occasion. She dreams of the lovely white 'standing out dress', standing out because of the stiff slip worn underneath. Then there's the beautiful toeless and heelless sandals, the delicate lace veil, the flower bouquet and the fragile cross and chain.

I'm looking forward to my big day, dreaming about it constantly, until my mother tells me that I can't have a standing out dress. It wouldn't suit me because of my leg. My left leg is the colour of a partially ripened plum and is much thinner and shorter than my right leg. I can't have the toeless and heelless sandals either because I will have to have a shoe that supports my foot.

And I will have to make do with my sister's communion dress, but now my heart's no longer in it. My shoes are closed in and though they are white with a little white button, I do not like them. Worse still, on the morning of my First Holy Communion, I find that the shoes are crippling me. I think that I will never get to the church. The only bonus is that on this occasion I can dispense with the heavy black boots and callipers for a few hours, even though walking is difficult and fraught with the danger that I will fall over if anyone merely brushes against me. But the teachers ensure that I'm given sufficient space and the event passes without mishap.

I am a picture of innocence, all in white, with a bunch of white lilies and white roses. But when the photographer places me under a tree and asks me to smile, I can see nothing to smile about. He tries everything, poor man, to make me smile. But I'm not having any of it. Eventually he sticks out his tongue and a glimmer of a smile passes my lips, but only because I think he looks so silly.

Because all the children making their First Communion have been fasting from midnight, a communion breakfast is laid on at the school. But I cannot eat anything. I am much too shy. In front of me are plates of buns and sweets and all the things that a poor child like me will not see again for a while. But I just can't eat.

Fearing that I will collapse, the teacher asks my mother to take me home and give me something to eat there. I am allowed to take a souvenir horseshoe-shaped stick of rock and that is the sum total of what I get.

The rest of the day is spent showing myself off to the neighbours and relatives, and more importantly collecting the money which is the rightful due of a first communicant.

***

At home at this time, a momentous event occurs. Modern technology, in the guise of a radio, comes to our house. It's a very large radio in a polished wooden case. The front has a large cloth-covered area with a round, brown knob on the left-hand side and a tiny little window on the right. Below this is a piece of coloured glass with two further knobs at either end. Behind the glass are vertical rows of printed words and a vertical red line that moves along behind the glass when the right-hand knob is turned.

When my father turns the left-hand knob, a light comes on behind the glass and a light comes on in the little window. Now the window appears to have curtains and when he turns the right knob the curtains open and close. It's magical and I want to play with it but we children are forbidden to touch the radio under pain of death. As this warning comes from my father and not my mother we well know from previous experience that it's an order that must be obeyed at all costs.

So we all stand around and stare at the radio while my father operates the knobs. Voices and music come from it and this I can't understand. I know there has to be people inside it. But how can even one person fit in there, never mind all of the Gallowglass Ceilí Band? It isn't even big enough for me to get inside it.

Maybe only their heads are in there and their legs are hanging out the back. I have a look around the back but it's blocked up and so I remain confused.

Some months later the light behind the glass doesn't come on and a man comes out from the shop to fix it. He removes the back while Charles Mitchell is reading the news. I realise this is my chance to have a look at him.

While the repair man is rummaging in his bag, I climb up on a chair and look in at the back of the radio. But all I can see is a round thing, like a large black bowl, and lots of little light bulbs and wires.

The voice is coming from the bowl and I am more baffled than ever. Now it seems that Charles Mitchell is in there. Maybe he can make himself very tiny and can then squeeze into that round bowl. I don't solve the puzzle until some years later, we get a television and I see for myself that all the people in Téléfís Éireann are only two inches tall.

***

In 1959 there is another momentous happening – I am officially declared handicapped, whatever that is. I know it has something to do with horseracing and also with golf. Golfers actually boasted about their handicaps, although it did appear that a 'one' handicap was better than a 'ten', though I couldn't imagine anyone being that handicapped, and still being able to play golf.

Being officially handicapped has its advantages, even though I still haven't got my number. First of all, I'm invited to a celebratory party in a local hall. I find that all the other children there are much worse than me. There is certainly no one under a 'ten'. I really feel a freak.

During the party we play musical chairs. I don't win though. I don't have the heart to push severely disabled children off their chairs. But one little brat, who is at least a 'twelve', thinks nothing of pushing me roughly to the ground. I learn a valuable lesson that day. The meek may not really get to inherit the earth, but they certainly get to spend a great deal of their time lying prostrate on it.

The other advantage of being officially declared handicapped – though still without a number – is that I get to make my trip to Knock. And though I go with hope, I return instead with wisdom and acceptance of my situation. Both are attributes I will need in the coming years if I am to continue to survive in a world that, unknown to me, has many more challenges ahead.

5

Hungry for Knowledge

❧

In 1960 I leave the 'babies' and go on to a bigger National School. It is a brand new building with highly polished floors. There are hairy tiles leading from the stairs to the door that opens onto the yard outside. We are not allowed to walk on the polished floor but must keep to those hairy tiles

The banisters on the stairs are gleaming, but they are not for holding onto while one climbs up and down. They are not a safety feature – not even to prevent disabled children like me from toppling down the stairs. They are for polishing and decoration and the only time they will be touched is when they are being polished. Certainly no tiny child's hand will ever touch them. And if it should do so, even accidentally, a much larger hand will strike fear and pain into that unfortunate child.

But the school has some advantages. It is much closer to home than the 'babies school' and also nearer than St Mary's Convent School, which my older sister Kathleen attends. She will continue going there as she has already settled in and is used to it. So once again I find myself alone.

To make matters worse, on my first day in this new school, I get off to bad start with the teacher, Miss Curtin. The girl who is seated behind me has the same name as me. She drops her pencil case which falls just beneath my desk. It is much nearer to me so I pick it up and hand it back to her.

'Thanks,' she says.

'That's OK,' I say. Our exchange can't even be described as a conversation. But the teacher shouts out the name I share with this girl behind me. 'Joan Ryan!'

I pay no attention to her. After all, I never get into trouble. No one stands up, so she repeats the name. Her voice is getting louder and louder and all the time I wonder why the girl behind me will not stand up. Eventually the teacher points at me. 'Joan Ryan,' she bellows. 'Stand up.'

Puzzled, I do so. 'You,' she says angrily, 'you were talking.'

'No, miss,' I protest, disconcerted by this false accusation.

The perceived lie enrages her. 'Come out here,' she screams.

I emerge from my desk, the centre of attention. All around me I can sense the malicious pleasure of my classmates at my discomfiture. I limp up to where she stands at the top of the room. 'Stand in the corner,' she orders, pointing with her finger, 'and face the wall.'

I have already learnt that authority cannot ever be openly questioned or challenged. There is nothing for it but to do as I am ordered. So I go and stand in the corner facing the wall, my back to the class for the rest of the morning. I am very hurt and deeply humiliated at this treatment, particularly as my mother has already explained to the head nun that I will not be able to stand for very long.

There is also the added humiliation of knowing that this is where the dunces stand in all the books I have read. I am only missing the cone-shaped hat with the letter D on it to complete my humiliation. But I will make my protest at this injustice in the only way I know. And that is to remain silent.

When eventually Miss Curtin asks me a question I do not answer. In silence I go on facing the wall with all the pent-up anger and frustration of a child who has been wronged. I am determined that this teacher will not get away with this unjustifiable act of cruelty. She will learn that I will never cower down – that she can thrash me or threaten all she likes, yet still I will remain silent.

Each time a question is put to me, I refuse to answer. When I am eventually told to return to my desk, I ignore the order. I don't even look around. Behind me I sense that Miss Curtin is getting more and more infuriated. She has got herself into a no-win situation and can do no more to me. I smile inwardly on detecting her anger and frustration.

When it is lunch time I decide that I've made my point and can now emerge from my corner. As I pass Miss Curtin on my way out of the classroom, she attempts to slap me on the behind. But I anticipate this and I take evasive action. I leave the classroom triumphant.

When I get home I tell my mother that I never want to go to that school again. Then the next day I pretend to be sick. I am determined that Miss Curtin will not get the better of me. I will not go to school ever again. I do not realise, of course, that this is not possible and that the law has other ideas. I will have to go to school whether I like it or not.

It is also the law at home. And while my mother will tolerate me being absent for one day, even if she suspects that I am not really ill, she will not continue to tolerate it. I also come to realise that I cannot pretend to be sick forever, particularly as my mother will not let me out to play when school is over. As far as she is concerned, being sick means being sick for the whole day.

So there is nothing for it but to accept my fate. I know that school is essential for me. I will have to learn and I will have to do well there. It has been instilled into me time and time again that I am different to the others in the family. I will always be different. It is vitally important that I do well at school because due to my handicap, I will not be suitable for many of the jobs which are usually available to girls from our background and education – jobs in factories and shops and cafés and hospitals and even as domestics in private houses.

So I swallow my pride and return to school. As I love learning and am normally eager and responsive, it is no time at all before Miss Curtin, to her credit, gets to know how to handle me. All she has to do is praise me and I will go to the moon for her. But if I am accused in the wrong or have any undeserved punishment meted out to me, then I will stay at home for days at a time. Even when I eventually return, I will remain silent while I am there. Gradually there develops a mutual respect between pupil and teacher.

I find that learning is easy for me. I hunger for knowledge and cannot wait to move on to the next pages in my English or Irish text book. I love arithmetic too and excel at mental arithmetic. I become proficient in every subject but knitting or sewing. They are to be my Achilles' heel.

I want to digest all the knowledge there is. I want to know everything about everything. But because of poverty, the tools I need, like copies and pens and ink and pencils, are almost impossible to obtain. The school provides free books for the poor children, but all the other necessities have to be provided by the parents.

One day I find that I need a new copy but my mother cannot afford the threepence to buy it. Yet how can I to go to school the following day without my exercises done? Apart from the fact that I always have my exercises done, it will mean two very hard slaps with a big stick for something that I have no control over.

I beg and plead for the threepence, but it's no use. My mother cannot produce money she just doesn't have. My sister Kathleen tries to console me. She is older and much more used to going without than me. She tells me the story of how when she went to her new school, she too had no copy and my mother tore open a brown paper bag and gave it to her to do her sums.

When she went to school the next day, the nun gave her four slaps and didn't even look at the work. My mother was very angry and immediately put pen to paper and wrote to the nun saying she could not afford a copy, and that if the nun had bothered to take the time to look at Kathleen's work, she would have seen that it was correct and that she was an intelligent child. No child, my mother wrote, deserved four slaps for being poor. That evening, before she left the school, Kathleen was given a free copy by the nun.

But I am not my sister. I know that I will not be brave enough to do my homework on a brown paper bag, not even if it were a posh brown paper bag. I need to see the blue ink standing out stark and clear against the white page. I need to see my sums all lined up neatly. I need lots of stars on my copy. No, I cannot go to school without my exercises completed in a copy, and I cry and cry until my mother relents and buys one on tick at the local corner shop. A lifetime later, I still feel guilty about that and realise why I am disliked by my family for the things I did as a child.

We have to have jotters too for school, but as they are for rough work, I am not as fussy about them. Any sort of plain sheets in a pad will do for jotting things down on. I am lucky that I don't have to buy these as my father brings lots of them home after a day out trying to earn some money. The teacher must wonder who this Pat Hogan, Turf Accountant is. If she asks, I will tell her that he is my father's accountant, only we have no money. The accountant has it all.

Hungry for knowledge, as I am, I want to know all there is to know about the world. I find that it annoys me intensely if something I learn at school does not concur with what I have already learned at home. I know that someone has to be wrong and someone has to be right – only I don't ever want to be the person who is wrong.

This trait is soon tested to the limit when a girl enters our classroom with a very important message for our teacher. When the girl leaves, the teacher announces in a very solemn voice that Sr Aquinas, our head nun, is engaged with Fr Griffin, and they are not to be disturbed.

Immediately my mind goes into overdrive. Did I hear correctly or has that girl got the message wrong? I can't believe what I've heard. Nuns and priests can't get married, yet here was the head nun announcing her engagement. It just doesn't bear thinking about.

But as they aren't afraid of telling people, maybe it's all right. Maybe they can't marry ordinary people who are usually terrible sinners, but can marry each other. That surely is the answer to the riddle. It's all very confusing. I cannot concentrate on my lessons – my mind is working overtime. I can't wait to get home and confront my mother with this news. When at last the bell rings I run all the way home and entering the house, gasping for breath, blurt out to my mother, 'I thought that nuns and priests couldn't get married?'

'Well they can't either,' she says.

'Well,' I say, 'Sr Aquinas has just got engaged to Fr. Griffin.' I am greatly relieved to get that off my chest.

'Ah no,' she says, 'you must have got it wrong.'

'No I haven't.' I'm adamant. 'She even sent a girl round to tell the whole school.'

My mother insists I am mistaken and I think to myself, 'You wait and see.' But Fr Griffin and Sr. Aquinas never do get married. I am not surprised because Sr Aquinas has many more engagements after that. In fact some of them are with other nuns! This is too scandalous to mention to anyone, never mind bringing it to the attention of my mother.

One of the advantages of the new school is that we are allowed out for drill, the forerunner of PE. This entails synchronised skipping around the yard. As I can only skip on one leg, I am not in sync with the other children and so I am made to sit on the wall. It is cruel as I can skip better on one leg than they can on two. Yet there I am, possibly the only child in the school who needs exercise, and I am sitting on the wall.

It is here that I first become a thinker. And I don't even have to take off my clothes like Rodin's man. As I place my hand on my chin, I wonder what the sun is made of and why are all the children skipping around the yard when they could be inside learning, and couldn't I have been sent home. That way, at the very least, I would get some exercise just by walking, and walking is supposed to be good for me.

After school we all have jobs to do at home. Life is hard on a woman with seven children in the house and everyone has to play their part. Life is also hard on the children, but we don't notice that. We don't worry about ordinary things like food and rent and electricity and coal. All we worry about is when can we get this stupid work done and go out to play.

There is no washing machine or hot water in our house, in fact no modern convenience whatsoever. Everything has to be done manually and it is all hard work. The only convenience available to my mother is the seven children to help with the work.

My job is to make the beds and sweep the bedroom floors. Because of my stays in hospital and the training I received there, I can make a bed as well as any nurse. I can tuck in the corners precisely. In fact it's child's play with sheets or blankets to work with, but quite another matter trying to tuck in, neatly or otherwise, the awkward shapes of coats.

Not that we have sheets either, though at times we are lucky enough to have sheets made from flour bags, only they are hard and coarse. At least they are better than a hairy blanket against the skin which causes one to continually scratch.

We are lucky indeed if we have one sheet to each bed. We also have maybe one rather tattered and worn blanket. The remainder of the bedding is made up of coats. And they are in plentiful supply. You would be forgiven for thinking we have a whole army of men at our house with the amount of coats we possess. There are at least three heavy ones to each bed.

I love neatness and, depending on how fast I want to get out to play, will reflect on how good the bed looks. Sometimes though, I just throw the clothes on the beds and sweep the bit of floor that can be seen before I rush out. More often than not though, I am dragged back in to do the beds properly.

My mother doesn't usually look under the beds and so the dust gathers there quietly until it becomes so high she can't help but see it. Then I'm in trouble and I have to do the job properly. As I sweep up, I begin to sneeze, and it continues all the while I am there. But no one takes any notice of a mere sneeze or two. There will be consequences though.

***

I am regarded as a big girl when we get the summer holidays and I am allowed to go to the cinema with my sister Kathleen for the first time. My father, for some reason, has been left minding us so he gives Kathleen the money to take us to see a film and get us out from under his feet. It is tuppence to gain entry to the local flea pit which passes for a cinema and this is meant to be a great treat for me. I am very apprehensive about going but Kathleen assures me it will be very funny. Yet it isn't. In fact, it's downright dangerous.

For a start it's pitch black in there and there are men shouting and fighting with one another at the other end of the building. I don't want to go in but Kathleen assures me again that it's just the film that's making all the noise and that I will be all right.

I trust her and follow her to our seats. But I have only just sat down when a very ugly and angry man points a gun straight at me. 'If you know what's good for you,' he says to me in a threatening voice, 'then you'll get out of town before sundown.' But as I can hardly see my sister, never mind the sun, I am up from my seat and out of there like a greyhound before I'm shot.

I don't even look behind me to see if I'm being followed by the man with the gun. My sister follows me, whispering threateningly that I'd best come back. But she can only come after me as far as the two swing doors. If she ventures outside, she will not be able to get back in. So she lets me off.

Kathleen berates me later for being so silly. 'It was only the film,' she says. 'You were perfectly safe.' It was difficult to believe that at the time though. It will be a while before I will venture to the cinema again.

6

Hard Times

ℭ℈

I love the summer. Most days seem sunny, and on those seem-ingly endless sunny days most of the children from the street walk out to the metal bridge. Here, it is claimed, the Shannon is 40 feet deep at the very centre of the river. It's a very dangerous spot, but most of the children don't seem to think of danger.

I never go in swimming, though almost all the other children do. Poverty is one reason why I don't go in – I don't possess a swim suit. Self-consciousness is the other reason. I am only too aware of the stares I will draw from the other children if I let them see my purple-blue leg. And there is also the fear of drowning. So I just paddle in the shallows close to the bank and watch the oth-ers swimming and splashing, the boys showing off, as usual.

I am even more terrified of crossing the metal bridge than venturing into the water. This bridge carries the railway line and the floor consists of just the wooden sleepers and boards in between, the river visible between the gaps, and the water seem-ing to be a very long way down.

The trains constantly use the bridge, so if you're on the bridge when one comes along, there are boxes along the sides you can slip into in order get out of the train's path. But they are so close to the rails, and therefore to the passing train, I don't have the courage to ever risk crossing to the other side.

One day, my eldest brother Tom offers to take myself and

Celia across the bridge. Encouraged by his age and by his assurances that I will be all right, I agree to go with him. I gingerly hop from one sleeper to the next, Tom comforting me when I get really scared halfway across and fear that I won't be able to go forwards or back.

But we make it to the other side and with his good deed done for the day, he goes in for a swim. Immensely proud of him, I watch him swim across what I know to be the longest river in the British Isles. He swims the whole width of the river, which to me seems a great distance.

Celia and I watch him get out on the other side, seeming to have shrunk on the way across. What if he is not coming back? I think. What are we to do, left here all alone and afraid? A young boy nearby senses our fear. It gives him an opportunity to taunt us and it is not an opportunity to be missed.

'He's not coming back,' he tells us. 'He'll just go on home and leave you both here. Then you'll never be able to cross the river and you'll never get home again.' We begin to cry with terror, not realising that Tom needs to rest on the other side before he can swim back to us.

The tears and terror ease when we see him start to make the journey back to us. As he draws nearer to the bank we dry the tears and put on brave faces. Our malicious tormentor makes himself scarce, aware of what might happen to him if we tell Tom what he did to us. But we remain silent, having learned a few salutary lessons: there are people in the world who only want to hurt you and one day you will have to face the world alone.

***

In the summer there are long days for playing on the street. But the days are not long enough and it is always annoying for us to be called in for supper. We possess only a few chairs. There is always a fight for the right to the few chairs which remain when my mother and father have sat down.

I have my own special small chair, but it is much too low for sitting at the table. Despite this, no allowances are made for me and more often than not, I am left standing.

It is the same story with the knives and forks and spoons. There are not enough to go around. Again, it's a matter of waiting for someone else to finish, otherwise one has to resort to using a spoon and it is very difficult to eat a soggy lettuce leaf with a spoon.

Our cups, when we have them, rarely have handles. Gradually they get broken and when this happens they are replaced by jam jars. I can never figure out where we get the jam jars as we rarely have jam. The jars somehow seem to keep the tea very hot and it always tastes delicious from them. There is one drawback though. It is difficult to drink the tea because, of course, the jam jars don't have handles and the glass gets very hot. So you have to pull the sleeves of your jumper down over your hands to pick up the jar.

There is little preparation for the return to school after the holidays. There is no money available to spend on preparations. The only thing that happens at this time of the year is the dispensary provides dockets for two pairs of free boots for the family. These are what we call 'boys' boots'. They are black, with a ribbon design going across them and no self-respecting person would willingly be seen dead in those ugly monstrosities.

But whatever about being a boy having to wear them, being a girl and having to wear them is the worst punishment that could ever be meted out. Because there are six in contention for the boots (I already have my horrible, special boots) and only two pairs of boots are allocated each year, this means that whoever got the boots the previous year, have to make do with the old ones.

The year old, or two-year-old boots usually have holes in them. These are blocked with brown paper to keep the rain out. Socks too will inevitably have holes in them, especially at the heels and toes. Clever people with no money who have holes in the toes of both the boots and socks polish their toes black to match the boots so that no one will be aware of the problem.

All too soon the holidays are over and I am back at school where our first task is to clean and polish our desks. It is hard work. 'Use some elbow grease,' the teacher encourages us.

We don't have uniforms in our school and the better-off girls are constantly trying to impress us less-fortunate ones with their expensive clothes. Teachers and pupils alike admire them. Most of my clothes – indeed most of my brothers' and sisters' clothes – are hand-me-downs, and always seem to come from kind people who just happen to be bigger than us and have no taste.

The clothes are always too baggy or too long or too flowery or too stripy. But our parents are glad of them, as it is one expense they are spared. I have a stroke of luck though and, much to my delight, get something to wear that is in vogue. It is the type of skirt that any girl would kill for – a real kilt.

I don't know if it is a Scottish or an Irish kilt. In fact I wouldn't care if it were an English kilt, if there is such a thing. All I know is that a kind neighbour is getting rid of some of her children's clothes and gives them to us. The real kindness here is that the clothes are still in good condition and have not yet gone out of style.

So I get a brand new, second-hand kilt from this act of generosity. At least to me, used to well-worn hand-me-downs, this kilt is brand new. It is beautiful, red plaid with a large silver pin to keep it closed. The skirt is pleated on one side, and straight at the other. I have always dreamed of having a pleated skirt, and though this one is only half pleated, nevertheless I am thrilled.

I realise that there isn't much point in having a pleated skirt if you cannot see the pleats. So I put it on with the pleats to the front and the plain part with the pin to the back. I'm told I have it on back to front but will I listen? No, not me. I'm adamant that I'm in the right.

So off to school I go, delighted with my new skirt. And luck is still on my side, for of all the teachers, in all the classrooms, in all the schools, in all the world, mine just happens to be wearing an almost identical skirt. But she is wearing it back to front. And she's supposed to be teaching me!

A cheeky pupil remarks to the teacher that my skirt is the same as hers and the teacher requests that I show it off properly to the class. It is almost certainly the first time the teacher has seen me in anything half decent. So I limp to the top of the class and then with encouragement from the teacher, clamber up onto her desk to show off my skirt to the best advantage.

I don't know how I manage to get up on that desk, but driven by the need to show off and gain the adulation I crave, I manage it.

And so I make my modelling debut, standing on top of the teacher's desk, elated by my good fortune and much relieved that I had the intelligence to put my skirt on the right way round. Maybe the other kids think I am being humiliated, but I lap up the attention. Ignorance really is bliss.

***

As the weeks pass I find I am progressing well at school and I like most subjects. But then when knitting and sewing become part of the curriculum I learn the meaning of terror. The running stitch is easy enough and I am delighted with the praise I receive when I show it to the nun. I can't wait to finish the felling bit so that I can go up and receive some more praise. But I cannot figure it out – no matter how hard I try. So with all the ripping out my blue piece of cloth is filthy. The only clean bits are the holes. The nun is disgusted and gives me such a thump on the back that I am sent running down the classroom and almost fall. It's only then I realise why it's called the run and fell seam.

I return home from school that day, praying, yet another time, that I won't ever have to go there again. And to my utter delight my prayers are instantly answered. My mother has had a letter from the Taoiseach asking if I could return to the hospital in Croom.

The letter is signed by Mr. Lemass himself. I know Mr Lemass is the Taoiseach, the head of the Irish Government, and here he is writing about me! Mise le Meas, it says at the end of the letter and I know enough Irish to know now that *Mise le meas* means I am Lemass, only I think it funny that the Taoiseach can't spell his own name correctly. But what do I care about that when he has taken the trouble to write about me?

A few days later I am off to the hospital in Croom. An ambulance calls for me – no fuss this time about my not being a Hungarian or a refugee. But then, with the Taoiseach personally intervening in my case, I couldn't expect anything less.

As I'm about to leave, Mrs Fitz, our neighbour, arrives with a sixpenny bar of Van Houten chocolate. It is the first time I have had a full bar of chocolate and I keep it in my hand and gaze at it regularly to ensure that I'm not simply dreaming. Another neighbour gives me six penny bars which, I feel, will last me forever. It is amazing the treats you get when God is on your side.

7

Getting the Boot

☙

After what seems a long and bumpy journey, I arrive with my mother at the Orthopaedic Hospital. Sister Dolan takes particulars at a desk and then my mother prepares to leave. I am about to get emotional at our parting when she leans down and kisses me on the cheek – a peck, nothing more. But I am acutely embarrassed by this. We don't have any such show of affection at home. I am seething and can't wait to see her again to tell her that she is never to behave like that again.

I am then given a bath. This is a real treat as we have no bath at home, just an enamel basin that we all get washed in on Saturday night. The basin is placed in front of the fire and we all stand in it and get washed. But, of course, you can't immerse yourself in a basin. So it is really wonderful to have a bath and lie submerged in the warm, soapy water.

After the bath, I am asked if I have slippers and a night-dress. Of course, I don't and it is embarrassing to have to say no. But they are used to this at the hospital. I am not the only poor child they will have dealt with.

They give me a rough flannelette night-dress that has already adorned the bodies of many other little girls, and I wonder if any of them were like me. Though rough, it feels lovely and clean and fresh. Properly dressed, I am taken along to a ward and shown to a bed. I can see immediately that it has sheets and I can hardly wait to just lie on those crisp white sheets.

Oh, the joy and the pleasure of it when eventually I slide down between the sheets. It is wonderful! I decide that I never want to go home again. I want to stay in this clean, fresh, sterile place forever.

And it gets even better. There are real meals too: breakfast, dinner and supper. I get a whole boiled egg in the morning and with my very own spoon. No waiting around for someone else to finish. There is jelly and ice cream after dinner and tasty sausages for tea. Hospital, I decide, is the most wonderful place in the world. Where else would a nine-year-old child from Killeely get such food? And to make life perfect, there is no full-time school, just occasional visits from a teacher, and therefore, no more terror of the run and fell seam to be endured. Mr Lemass has done a perfect job. God will be very pleased with him. And even if I don't know why I'm here, I am beginning to understand why people might break a leg to get in here.

After a few days I really begin to enjoy myself. It is great here because I am not sick. But strangely, I am missing home, which puzzles me. I am also missing having some sweets, not that we had very many when I was at home. One always had a friend though, who might give you a bite of whatever they had when they were feeling generous, or just a lick if they were feeling mean. Even a lick of a toffee bar, when your tongue is hanging out for something sweet, is the most delicious and satisfying feeling in the world. But I have no sweets here. The bar of chocolate and the six penny bars are gone.

Most patients have a little money, or they receive parcels from home with lots of goodies in them. Most are very kind and will share what they have. But I feel bad about taking their goodies when I never have anything to give back. Each day I hope that the postman will bring me something – even a letter – but he never does.

Many of the patients are confined to bed, but myself and one other girl are mobile. It is a great feeling and I exult in it. For the first time in my life I am the fittest and ablest person there. I can do anything I want and they can't catch me or punish me. Charles Darwin would have been proud of me. He could have written about this new species that could change and learn to adapt itself to its new environment. This was no desert, no Galapagos Islands – this was Croom Orthopaedic Hospital, but the fight for survival still goes on.

Power corrupts even nine-year olds. Normally a very shy introvert, I become extroverted and bask in the glory of adulation. One night the girl opposite me asks if I would like a sweet. Would I like a sweet? This is surely the understatement of the year. I am desperate for something sweet, having spent weeks in here without access to sweets of my own.

Yet at this moment I am more than willing to travel eleven miles; I will willingly climb a mountain; I will sweep the sugar off the floor in a sweet factory; I will do anything for a sweet. Well, not quite anything. I won't go back to the run and fell seam for a start. Yet I don't want the girl to see how desperate I am, so I say, 'Well OK. Yes, please.'

'Well you'll have to come over for it,' she says.

I stare at the floor. The tiles are shiny and look cold. I know it must be cold as it is now late October. I have no slippers and my toes tingle imagining the cold of the tiles. 'Can you throw it over?' I ask. 'I don't want to go out on the cold floor.'

'OK,' she says. She really does try, but she isn't up to Olympic standards and the sweet falls on the floor about a foot out from the end of her bed. There it sits, tempting me to come and get it. It has to be picked up from there anyway, otherwise someone with two good legs might slip on it and end up in here with us cripples.

'What are you going to do now?' she asks. A sweet sitting on the ward floor is an insurmountable problem for anyone confined to bed. But I am the King of the Castle. I am the only one here capable of removing this sweet from the floor.

'I'll get it,' I say.

'How?' she asks. 'You'll have to walk on the cold floor now.'

'No, I won't,' I say. 'I'll just jump across to your bed.'

'But you can't do that,' she says.

'Of course I can,' I boast. 'It's simple. I'll just stand up here on the end of my bed and jump across.'

She is in awe now and so are the other patients. I am thrilled. I have an audience and I have to entertain them. I place my right foot on the top rail of the iron bed end and then, gripping it with both hands, haul myself up until I'm in a crouched position and balanced unsteadily. I then bring my left leg up and place it on the top of the rail. Gripping the rail with my toes and using my hands, I push myself into a more upright crouch. I release my left hand and, using it to balance myself, begin to rise further. When I'm at the extremity of my right-hand reach, I release that too. Now, using both hands, arms outstretched, and taking all the weight on my right leg, I slowly stand upright, wobbling precariously, disaster and broken limbs, or worse, waiting four feet below me on those cold, shiny, hard tiles.

Still wobbling, but balancing as best I can with my arms outstretched, I prepare myself for the great Evel Knievel leap across to the other bed. It is a yawning chasm, the Grand Canyon itself, but surely twice as wide and with twice the drop to disaster.

It is while I am imagining my leap across that vast space, and standing poised to make it, that the sister comes into the ward. I catch her entrance out of the corner of my eye and take a deep breath, certain now that I'm in serious trouble. But to my utter surprise and disbelief, she begins to clap loudly. I am thrilled and delighted with her approbation and to impress her even more stand on my good right leg.

It is then she screams. This causes me to lose my concentration and I sway wildly before toppling backwards onto the bed. She is furious and charges towards my bed, her face glowing red and her eyes seemingly on fire. 'How dare you?' she screams. 'How dare you do such a stupid thing? Get back under the bed clothes at once.'

This seems a superfluous order, as I am desperately trying to do just that. There is a hush of expectation all about the ward but I can sense the fear from the other patients too. A sister on the rampage, just like a teacher, is likely to vent her spleen on anyone, even the most innocent of all.

I somehow manage to scramble beneath the bedclothes, no pleasure now to be gained from crisp clean sheets. 'If you dare budge out of there again,' the sister continues to threaten, 'I'll have you tied to the bed with chains.'

I'd learned by now that I was in the hospital to be measured for a special shoe for my left leg. Once I'd got this shoe I could dispense forever with the horrible black boots and callipers. But here they were now, treating me as if I were a prisoner in a chain gang. Maybe at this rate I'd end up with a big ball and chain attached to the shoe as well.

My moment of glory is replaced with tears and fears. And I have no sweet either for my pains. But was my bit of glory worth it? Of course it was! For one minute I basked in adulation.

Yet there is a price to pay for everything and that night I pay my price. I cry myself dry in the dim light which illuminates the ward, and with fear coursing through my body, my bladder, weak at the best of times, seems to weaken even more. I am too terrified to get out of the bed to go to the toilet. And in the distance I'm certain I can hear the clanking as they get the chains ready for me, just in case.

I try to control my bladder but it is hopeless and I end up wetting the bed. As Joyce points out, obviously from previous experience, first it is warm and then it gets cold.

It causes me to wriggle and squirm and brings a rather large and terrifying nurse to my bedside to see what is the matter. She knows from experience what the problem is, but changing a child's wet sheets in the middle of the night is not hospital policy. Presumably to save on laundering costs, a wet sheet – particularly if one had only wet a small bit of it – is not replaced. It is removed entirely. Then the nurse simply takes the top sheet and folds it over so that it is both under and over the patient. This is what is called a 'fresh' bed.

Now this is fine where the patient is a small child. Their legs will barely reach the fold. And anyway, a child is probably expected to curl up their legs. I am a small child so everything should be all right. But I am uneasy. I am fidgeting. When I stretch out my legs, the longer right one comes up against the restriction of the fold.

I am mischievous, and like Wodehouse, if not exactly disgruntled, I am not terribly gruntled either. I suppose it is those two attributes that makes me act when I feel the pressure of the sheet against my foot. I thrust my foot hard at the fold again and again, venting my spleen on the street.

When I hear it rip and feel my leg shoot out into empty space, I know that I am in even more trouble. Now I spend the rest of the night in greater terror. In the morning I play the innocent and as if to make up for my rash act of standing on the end of my bed, I give the nurses a great hand making the beds in the morning. I strip my own bed myself, bundle up my torn sheet and throw it in the laundry basket. Only then can I relax, aware that I am safe for the moment.

Even at nine years of age I take modesty in dress very seriously. Yet despite my innate modesty and at such a tender young age too, I have to wear a G-string. Just a G-string and nothing else – a green one to boot and it isn't even St Patrick's Day. Despite this, I still have to parade around in it. Give me the ball and chain any day.

So here I am, minus harp, shamrock and music, marching up and down the ward while the sister, a nurse and a doctor in a white coat stares at me.

I am mortified at this parade. There is certainly no glory to be had here. Eventually a 2" piece of cork is attached to the sole of my left foot and, hey presto, everyone is smiling. I am cured! The doctor winks at me and pats me on the leg.

The special shoe which will now be made for me, I'm assured, will change my life. Everyone is excited at this prospect. But two long weeks are to pass before it arrives. Meanwhile, I feel like Cinderella waiting for my prince to come with the glass slipper. I had lost out for my communion in not being able to have the sandals I wanted, but now I will have the perfect shoe.

When it does arrive, it fits perfectly. But horror of horrors, this is no dainty slipper. And instead of feeling like a princess, I feel like the two ugly sisters all in one. My longed-for dainty shoe turns out to be another boy's boot. It is black and ugly and cumbersome, and feels as heavy as if it had two balls and chains attached to it. If they gave me a pair of crutches, I'd be much happier.

A few days later I see a pair of crutches behind the ward door. 'They must be for me,' I think, delighted at this unexpected turn of events. They are wooden crutches, beautifully polished. They even have a piece of rubber at the bottom to stop slipping. Able bodied people think they know it all. But they obviously don't know that disabled people never fall off their crutches.

I look longingly at them and when I think no one is looking, I decide to try them out. They are very tall and I have great difficulty trying to fit them under my arms. To the best of my knowledge, Tiny Tim never had this trouble. Whatever I do, I can't get them to stand up straight. And the rubber yolks at the end don't really do their jobs at all.

Eventually myself and the crutches crash to the floor. The whole ward's attention is riveted on me as I pick myself up, my face red from the humiliation. I retreat to my bed, convinced now that crutches mightn't be such fun after all.

Whether it's due to the episode with the crutches and a fear in the hospital that I will end up breaking my good leg before I leave or not, but the following day I'm told that I can go home. Days pass before an ambulance is available to take me.

Some days later an ambulance arrives and at last and I can go home. The driver doesn't know exactly where I live so I have to go into the front with him and show him the way, once we get to our local Church.

My mother is in town when I arrive home and the ambulance man doesn't want to leave me alone in the house. 'Where might your father be?' he asks me and I tell him that he's probably out with his accountant. That's where he usually is.

'Is there a neighbour I can leave you with?' he asks, and I tell him he can leave me with Mrs Fitz. She is only too delighted to see me home again, safe and well, and the ambulance driver goes off satisfied that I'm in good hands. But he is no sooner gone than I'm off down the street with my friends, regaling them with my adventures in the hospital. The poor ambulance man obviously doesn't know that street children don't need to be treated with kid gloves, not even lame ones like me, with big, black ugly boots.

8

WAR AND PEACE

෴

The boot curtails my movement almost as much as the calliper once did. In our street games of tag I am much too slow, and easily caught. But as the tagger, it's even worse. I can never tag anyone and soon my companions tire of the game and run off to some new adventure. I am left to follow them, asking them to wait.

A kind neighbour, as if moved by my efforts to drag the boot around with me, gives me the money to go with her daughter and friends to the circus. But I never get to see the circus. Crossing the green to the big top, I trip over a wire. By the time I scramble to my feet, I've lost my friends in the crowd. As I drag myself home, I promise myself that one day I will get to see the circus. Some day there will be someone to look after me, someone who will not rush off and leave when I stumble and fall.

A few days after my return from the hospital, I am back at school. It is hard going, dragging the big boot up the stairs. But the staff are very kind. They tell me that I can go to the end of the line so that I won't be holding everyone up and there will be little danger of anyone knocking me down. Most important of all though, I won't have to hold onto their pristine banister.

The big boot is the bane of my life. How I come to hate it. It really makes me feel a freak. And if I feel a freak, then I think that I must look like one. Freaks attract attention – the worst type of attention: the attention that ridicules without admiration; the attention that hurts without praise; the attention that one can very well do without.

Crossing the yard at school is a nightmare for me. I constantly worry that if someone bumps into me, I will fall. Yet I am not afraid of getting hurt, just that everyone will see my knickers.

Yet, as per Murphy's Law, it is inevitable that one day something terrible will happen. And inevitably it does. I am walking slowly across the yard, careful to avoid contact with all the other running, jumping, laughing children, when a group of boys decide to have some fun. There is only one class of boys in this all girls' school. These are the first-class boys.

It seems as if all of them descend on me at once, surrounding me with their chants, 'You're wearing boys' boots. Look, she's wearing boys' boots'. They have a rope, probably a skipping rope taken from a group of girls. They wrap the rope about my waist and race off across the yard, dragging me after them, as though I am a stubborn animal and this is the only way to get me to move.

I cannot run as fast as they can, and a terrible terror seizes me as they drag me along. I feel myself falling helplessly to the ground, the sky and the earth spinning about me. But before they can drag me along the ground, a girl in a higher class intervenes and stops the torture. To this day I still remember Delma Reidy with affection and gratitude.

As I raise myself up and Delma helps to undo the rope, I feel dazed and shocked. However I do not cry. I will not cry. No one will ever see me cry. I will have to be tough. I will have to be strong. Above all else, I will have to keep my feelings to myself.

I cannot concentrate for the rest of the afternoon. I remain silent, much to the annoyance of the teacher. But one of the girls explains that some boys have been bullying me. Bullying? Is that all it was – just bullying? There must be a stronger word than that to describe the incident. For me it was to experience sheer terror. It was torture. It was cruel. It was inhuman. From now on I decide that I will hate and detest boys. Indeed I vow always to hate and detest them.

But this incident is to be a turning point in my life. When I return home from school that day, the dreaded, hated and detested boot gets the boot. I pronounce in a loud determined voice, that I am never going to wear it again. Even my mother and father cannot reason with me. They point out that the boot is necessary – that I must wear it for my own good. Wearing it means that I do not limp. It also evens out my stance and so there will be no adverse affect on my spine if I continue to wear it. But I remain adamant. There will be no more boot for me.

What is the point in walking tall and straight and without a limp and then ending up getting battered because I'm wearing boys' boots, I reason? It will only be a matter of time before I end up limping with both legs if that goes on. Far better to limp naturally and not suffer the so-called bullying. As far as the family is concerned though, this irony is lost on them. As far as they're concerned, I am being bold and unco-operative, as usual. But I endure their approbation, knowing that they will never understand what I feel or the hurt I endure. From now on though, I will lick my wounds myself in isolation.

As if to add further irony to the whole situation, some weeks later I am summoned to the dispensary to be vaccinated against a dreaded disease. The nurse sits me on my mother's lap and asks what is wrong with my leg as she pricks me with the needle.

'She had polio,' my mother says.

'What!' the nurse exclaims. 'But I've just vaccinated her against it.'

Yippee! I think I've just got a polio injection. Lucky me indeed! That should keep me safe from the dreaded disease and the ignominy of having to wear a horrible boot on my other foot.

But there are worse things than polio to fear in the early months and years of the 1960s. It begins with the Bay of Pigs invasion and the so-called invaders returning without a sausage, never mind a nice bit of bacon. President John F. Kennedy is making threats against the Russians and the Cubans. A man called Khrushchev is thumping tables and strutting about with lots of frightened men running after him. In Cuba, Fidel Castro goes about dressed in a dirty uniform, a bushy beard, and with his hair uncombed.

There is fear everywhere that there is going to be a terrible nuclear war which will affect the whole world. A booklet is sent to every house in Ireland. It warns us to stay inside for months after the war, preferably under the stairs – all nine of us. I don't know what people without stairs will do – vaporise, I suppose.

We should also put bags of sand to the front and back doors. Apparently sand is your man to keep out the radiation. The booklet does not tell us where to get the sand, nor the bags. The only sand we know of is at the beach in Kilkee and we have never even been there.

The booklet also exhorts us to store plenty of tinned food – meat and beans and anything else that might be nourishing. I don't know where we are going to keep all those tins. They won't fit under the stairs with all of us. Anyway, I reckon the air outside would possibly be safer than what we could hope to gasp under the stairs after eating all those beans. I'm willing to take my chance with the radiation.

The war does not break out (at least not yet) and we don't have to huddle beneath the stairs with our beans. But despite the war not breaking out, I find myself seriously wounded. I have not been shot, I have not been stabbed. In fact, I haven't even been hit with a missile, never mind a nuclear one. But I am verbally wounded; no band aid will cure the hurt that has been inflicted on me.

I have been called a cripple. Imagine me, a cripple? Logically it can't be true. I should be wounded first, then crippled. But if I'm supposed to be a cripple, which I'm not, why is it that only now I feel wounded? I decide that the rotters who threw this insult at me are just plain stupid. They don't know what they are talking about. But just to be sure, to be sure, I decide to look it up in the *Oxford English Dictionary*. They should know things like that. I decide I will be thorough in my search though. I will look up not just the word cripple, but limp and lame too.

Extract from the *Oxford English Dictionary*:

'Limp: Walk lamely.' Well that's true enough. 'Of damaged ship, aircraft, etc.' Not applicable. I have nothing to do with ships or aircraft, not even with etc. 'Proceed slowly or with difficulty.' I'd never noticed that since I got rid of the big boot. 'Of verse – be defective.' Me! Never! I can recite *The Boy Stood on the Burning Deck* without even pausing for breath. 'Lame walk.' Well all right. I'll give it that one.

'Lame: Disabled by injury or defect especially in leg or foot.' Well as I was never injured, than I must be defect, whatever that is. But it sounds serious enough. The *Oxford Dictionary* isn't doing my self-esteem any good at all so far. 'Limping or unable to walk normally.' Not exactly true. I might not be able to walk properly, but I can certainly limp properly. 'Of excuse etc.' I don't know what that means but maybe they're only using it as an excuse to slip in that etc. again. 'Lame dog, Lame duck.' I'd never seen a duck limp, but I'd once seen a dog dragging his leg behind him. I neither bark nor quack though, so I'm safe there. 'Insolvent person.' Clearly someone who's been soaked in solvent, whatever that is. So that leaves me out for those last two definitions. 'Make lame; disable.' 'Gosh,' I decide, 'I must be much worse than I think.' After all the *Oxford Dictionary* cannot be wrong. And I still haven't got to the big one.

'Cripple: Permanently lame person.' Well, there it is in black and white and I'd never have believed it. It is terrible. According to the Oxford English Dictionary I am a cripple. How awful. I am a defect. How doubly awful. What can I do? Well, there is only one thing to do. I'll give the dictionary the Churchill Victory Sign. What do they know about me anyway, the foreigners? Next time I'll look up the 'Limerick Irish Dictionary'.

Despite the fact that I am now, according to the *Oxford English Dictionary*, a cripple, it doesn't prevent me getting the summer holidays from school. The great day arrives and still there is no war. It's just as well though because the days are long and sunny now, and it would be really hot and stuffy, not to mention smelly, under the stairs.

With so much spare time at home, my friend Theresa and I are constantly arguing with our parents. This is war of the domestic type. We are constantly bombarded with jobs which we don't want to do, particularly as the weather is glorious and we want to be outside, playing in the sunshine.

Because everyone is poor and money is in such short supply, we've always been encouraged to save what little we get. Even during the threat of war, we're encouraged, which is a mystery to me. Where are we ever going to spend the money if we're going to be hiding under the stairs? And even if we survive, the whole world will have been destroyed when we eventually come out. But knowing that parents are the most illogical people on earth, where money is concerned, it is as well to do as they bid.

It is a mystery to me where I get my money from, but I somehow am able to save a few pence every now and then. So along with Theresa, I have been saving sixpenny stamps in a post office saving's book. Some of the money comes from Theresa's father. Whenever he gives her a shilling, he gives me something as well. When full, the saving's book contains forty sixpenny stamps, equivalent to the princely sum of £1.00. One day, out of sheer frustration, we decide to draw all our saving out of the Post Office and spend it stupidly. That, we think, should upset our parents and show them what's what.

So off we go to the local sub-post office. The woman behind the counter there isn't very friendly. Maybe our little books are holding up the exchequer, whatever that is.

Theresa fills in her form very neatly and in very small figures writes the amount of withdrawal: £1.00. The post mistress takes the form and very aggressively writes £1.00 in big figures over Theresa's small figures. I am watching all this and think to myself that that is not going to happen to me. The tyrant won't have any reason for complaint. So when I come to fill in the amount, I write in great big figures £1.00, very adult, not a bit afraid to lean on the pen.

I hand the form to the lady behind the counter who takes it, looks at it and shouts: 'What's this? Sure you've only ten shillings in your book.' I'm afraid my friend and I get a fit of the giggles, but our friend behind the counter is not amused. I don't bother trying to explain what happened. She will never believe that I am simply trying to be perfect. Instead she will think that I am, in fact, trying to defraud the Post Office of ten shillings.

Anyway she gives us our money, which we wisely (or so we think) spend on sweets and chocolate, munching away happily for the rest of the day. But the hours of blissful chewing and sucking are followed by not only pains in our bellies, but toothache as well. And now we have no money left in the Post Office to boot. Still, the summer goes on.

The long days are spent skipping and playing games. It is great exercise after the confinement of school. They had drill there now and again, but I was never allowed to take part because I was a defect. Yet I can hop and skip and jump. It's dead easy because I've only got the one leg to worry about.

Life is never prefect though, and you can't ever win. If you can't skip you get ridiculed and hurt. If you can skip better than everyone else, then you also get ridiculed and hurt. Not hurt by physical blows, but by words. Words are the most hurtful of all weapons.

'Sticks and stones may break my bones, but names will never hurt me.' So goes the old saying, rattled off parrot fashion when someone is called a hurtful name. How many of us recite that while our hearts are breaking? If you ask me, sticks and stones and broken bones, though certainly physically painful, would do far less damage to the human spirit than any cruel words.

I am so good at hopping on one leg that it is inevitable that I should be hurt by words. This hurt is caused by my being identified with a literary villain. Naturally I am very upset by this. And while I wouldn't mind at all being called Short Joan Silver – especially if I also found my very own 'treasure island' – any able bodied, or indeed any disabled bodied seaman, would object strongly

to being called Hopalong Cassidy. Yet despite this cruel appella-
tion, I still skip on and I still out-do everyone else.

The hot weather, though, can't last forever and in August the
storms come and the river Shannon bursts its banks. The water
floods out onto the roads, and nearby houses have to be evacuat-
ed. While the adults wring their hands in despair, we children are
thrilled. The water is a wonderful attraction. It seems to stretch
for miles up the road and most children take off their shoes and
socks and venture in a little way.

Water is dangerous and everyone knows that the further in
you go, the deeper it will be. But because I am a genius, I know I
can walk the whole length of the flood – the water can only be the
same depth because the road here is flat. So I tell my friends that
I am going to walk through the whole flood, right to the end.

'You can't,' they say, both horrified and in awe.

'I bet you I can,' I say.

'How much?'

'A shilling.'

'OK.'

I remove my shoes and socks and enter the water. I know I am
cheating, but it doesn't matter because, as usual, I don't get away
with it. I know there are manholes along the road, but I don't
reckon on one not having a cover. As I walk along, cocky as can
be, I step on empty air and drop straight down like a stone, letting
out a merciless scream with the fright.

I have only fallen about a foot, but it might as well have been
twenty feet, such is the fright I've had. Yet worse than the fright
are the jeers and laughter of my friends once they recover from
the fright they've obviously had.

Defeated, humiliated, and knowing that I will have to face the
wrath of my mother (my wet dress will be a dead giveaway as to
what I have been up to) I'm forced to retreat. It's a lesson to me
not to be so cocky, and I do remember it for a day or two. But then
being me, I forget!

9

BROKEN BREAD

❧

The holidays end all too soon and we find ourselves back at school. Life becomes serious again. But we have our little interludes. One of these occurs when a ballet teacher comes to the school seeking out talent. There is a new ballet school starting up in the area and she is looking for recruits.

The ballet teacher is tall and elegant and beautiful. We don't often see people like that in our rough neighbourhood and I'm fascinated by her. I decide there and then that I want to be a prima ballerina. I want to be tall, and straight and elegant too. Ballet will be the making of me.

I practice standing on my toes for hours and hours. Indeed I find that I can stand on my toes wearing ordinary shoes, unlike the ballet dancers who have to have special shoes. And I just know that my left leg would stay raised right up if Rudolph Nureyev held it. In fact, anyone's leg would stay up if he held it.

I've seen him on the television in my friend's house. Despite being gorgeous and the best dancer in the whole world, he is seeking asylum. I decide that, mad or not, he can come round to our house any time and hide under the stairs with us.

I am fully confident I can be a ballerina, yet days later I have to face the awful reality that I will never ever succeed in my dream. And not because of polio, the dreaded Big P, but because of the lack of LSD. My parents cannot afford the pounds, shillings and pence for lessons. They cost as much in LSD as LSD itself. I can have no hallucinations about that. This dream is short lived, but there is no shortage of dreams. I may not make it as a ballet dancer but vow that I will be rich and famous one day.

In the meantime, there is always the ever-present poverty which prevents one from achieving their dreams. This is not so noticeable in the summer, when children can go barefoot, and indeed are expected to do so. The few rags of clothes we possess are light and can be easily washed and dried. Fires are not needed and there is hardly any need for electric light. So we survive and have fun.

There are also means of obtaining a few pennies or treats in kind like the visit of the ragman who comes down the road calling, 'Piles of aul rags! Piles of aul rags!' All the children scatter to their homes to look for rags. Our whole house is full of rags and it is a case of picking out the worst of those that can no longer be mended.

In exchange for these rags we are given a balloon and a piece of chewing gum, which is a great treat indeed. Because we are so poor, we do not have any luxuries, and it's up to ourselves to come up with ways and means of obtaining money. Children are much better at this than the adults, who are bowed down by the sheer harshness of life.

My older brother Pat is a real expert. How often he has kept us from cold and hunger I do not know? He is constantly trying to earn money. He collects bones and also saves the bones left over from our own dinner. These are mainly back bones, with the tail still attached and are usually the meat ingredients of a stew, though in fact there is very little meat on them.

When Pat has collected a bag of these bones he sells them to a local farmer. The stench from the bag is simply awful and, especially in the summer, one avoids the coal house where the bag is kept. I don't know what the farmer does with the bones and I do not want to know.

Pat also goes daily to the local dump where he collects

enough wood for the fire. Searching through the piles of rotting refuse, he also finds wine bottles, beer bottles, lemonade bottles – indeed all types of glass bottles. When he has filled his bag, he carries the great heavy load home on his back.

The bottles have to be washed, a most arduous task in freezing cold water in the winter time. When the bottles are clean and sparkling, he sells them on to a local man who deals in bottles. There is a twopence refund on most types of bottle and Pat gets half of that from the man.

Old electrical cables too are a good source of income. But there is a great deal of hard work involved in stripping the cable to reveal the shiny copper inside. When he has collected about a stone in weight, he then sells it to someone who deals in scrap metal. Whatever he gets from these enterprises – sometimes maybe as much as five shillings – he gives most of it to my mother. It helps to feed us for another day.

The dump is a fascinating place. Whenever I've been there I've been amazed by what people have thrown out. I wonder do they know that their rubbish is one of the means of our living and surviving.

One time it is rumoured that thousands of pounds have mistakenly been thrown out with the rubbish and there are more people than flies buzzing around the dump trying to find the money.

Children from the locality usually frequent the dump to see what can be found. Broken toys which can be mended are a strong attraction. One time we think we have struck it rich when we find thousands of dollars in confederate currency. Alas, it is of no value, but we still collect it and count it, wishing it were good.

Sweets and biscuits and all kinds of other edible goodies are regularly dumped but we are warned to never eat anything like that. No matter how tempting a sweet or biscuit might appear, it could be deadly poisonous. Yet many people make a living from the dump and even eat from it too.

One time we find a box of discarded gas masks and it's as if Santa Claus has come in the middle of summer. For weeks the children of the area go around wearing the masks and talking funny. Naturally, the boys play at being soldiers while we girls soon tire of the novelty and return to our skipping ropes or games of 'picky'.

Like almost everyone I know, I dread the winter because of the cold and damp. When it's raining and cold, it's hard to keep warm. The beds are piled with coats and this makes them very uncomfortable. But this has to be endured along with the hairy blanket which itches something terrible, and causes me to wake at night, terrified and breathless. One night the breathlessness is worse than usual. As I struggle to suck the air down into my lungs, it is Pat who runs downstairs and brings up his bottle of orange that he has worked so hard for. He gives it to me and I manage to gulp down some of it. With its fizzy tang and bite, the relief I feel as it slips down my throat will remain with me always.

We then get sheets when my mother obtains some flour bags She sews a number of bags together and makes a coarse type of sheet that ranks amongst the best of them. There is no such thing as fancy bed linen. Ranks Flour provides our sheets, and glad we are to have them. I hope that the sheets will prevent the hairy blanket from not only scratching me, but making me breathless as well, yet it turns out to be a forlorn hope. Over the years the breathlessness will only get worse.

There is still the bitter cold though, and when we complain about it, my mother advises us to put our feet into our jumper or cardigan. It will be warm straight from our bodies and we, in turn, will be nice and cosy. It works well and is a real treat.

There are three of us sharing the one bed and that too helps to keep warm, except, of course, when one of the others drag the bedclothes off me. There is more room for the three of us if two sleep at the top of the bed and one at the foot. Yet sleeping at the foot, there is always the danger of having one of the other two occupants' smelly toes stuck in your mouth.

But if keeping warm at night is a major problem, doing so during the day is a real nightmare. We don't have any warm coats

– despite the piles on the beds – and no scarves, gloves or warm shoes. So for the most part, it is the extremities – the hands, feet and face – that bears the brunt of the cold. We all suffer, but none more so than my older sister, Kathleen.

***

Kathleen attends St Mary's school because our new local National Girls' School had not yet been built when she left the infants' school. Once she had started at St Mary's, she didn't want to leave and return to the new school when it was built. I suppose she had her friends there and didn't want to leave them.

St Mary's is more than a mile from home and it is a long, cold walk on a wet winter morning or evening. But the fact that Kathleen goes there has one great advantage. Tubridy's bakery is quite near the school and on her way home, Kathleen's job is to get bread there. We cannot afford proper loaves so we get the broken bread. A bag costs one shilling and sixpence and we depend on it for a major part of our diet.

Sometimes there is no broken bread left, but we don't go hungry. A man who works there and who knows us and our situation, deliberately breaks the fresh bread for Kathleen. It is a simple act of true Christian charity, and so often the poor survive because of such acts of kindness. This man is probably risking his own livelihood in doing what he does and perhaps one might claim that it is sinful or wrong, or even illegal. But I prefer to see it as genuine Christian charity.

The fresh bread is always a rare treat because it tastes so nice. Normally we would get the old stale bread. So, day after day, Kathleen carries the bread home. In winter time she is often frozen to the marrow as she carries the bag and her school bag on the long journey home to Killeely.

One Saturday, on the way home with the bread, she meets my father. Because it's Saturday and there is no school, she has our baby brother, Buddy, with her and her bare hands are frozen from the steel handle of the pram. Dad places his own hands over hers and together they wheel the pram home. And the warmth she feels creeping into her hands is precious, because it is warmth generated by love. It must have been intense because to this day she can still feel the warmth of his hands on hers.

***

This year at school I am not alone. I have my very own body-guard and will no longer have to live in fear of the journey to and from school. I feel it's going to be brilliant. My sister, Celia, is joining me in the new school. But things don't always work out the way we might wish.

Mostly Celia runs off with her friend. Even she does not want to be seen with me. I am too slow, too timid, too afraid and too goody good. I never get into trouble. But then, I don't need to get into trouble. Trouble usually finds me.

I have no one to talk to or no one to understand my predicament. I am a child who is different – a so-called special child, only the special child is usually special because of her inability to stand up for herself. The very act provokes such a backlash that she learns quite quickly that she may as well do nothing. But I do something. I become moody, which doesn't endear people or family to me. I become silent when hurt, but they don't understand – they will never understand.

Often I am the innocent caught in the crossfire of someone else's misbehaviour, and one such occasion happens this school year. To add insult to injury, I wasn't even at school when the terrible deed which was to affect me so much, was done.

It was so bad that the children didn't even speak of it among themselves, no doubt terror stricken by the anger of the head nun, which is sufficiently potent to curdle blood. And the reason for all this, is the pristine banister, that even I am not allowed to hold either going upstairs or down, has been scratched.

Someone in the school – it has to be a pupil for no one else would be capable of such wickedness – has dragged something like a hair clip from the top of the banister right to the very bottom. It is a long deep scratch and stands out like a meandering river on a brown map. The whole school is suspect and everyone is asked if they have seen anyone do it.

The conclusion is that it had to be done when someone went to the toilet. All the children have to raise their hands and request in Irish: '*Bfuill cead agam dul amach, ma se do hoille*' which translated means: May I go out, please? I am too scared to ever raise my hand for anything except to answer a question, so there is no possibility that I can be responsible for this act of wanton vandalism.

The school has a policy that children with weak bladders or kidney problems don't even have to ask permission to go to the toilet. Having to listen to '*Bfuill Cead agam dull amach ...*' dozens of times a day is more than enough for any teacher to bear, never mind having to listen to it dozens of times from those regularly short taken. So the policy is to grant those pupils absence without leave.

There is a girl in my class who is allowed out at any time and my sister Celia, who is in a lower class than me, is also in this situation. When the head nun gets to Celia's class on her round of interrogation, she orders them all to kneel before a statue of Our Lady and to swear to tell the truth. Hellfire, she tells them, is beneath the floorboards. Any girl who doesn't tell the truth will fall into the fire when the boards part beneath her and down there she will burn forever with the Devil and all the fallen angels.

Under this threat, Celia tells the nun that she saw the girl from my class with the weak bladder dragging the clip down the banister. And so while Celia saves herself from the fires of hell, unknowingly, she inadvertently drops me right into them. But I know nothing of this. So when the culprit is punished for her terrible deed, we think that should be an end of the matter. And by the start of the new week it should be forgotten

On Sunday my father sends me for the paper. I am happy as I begin my return journey home, the newspaper tucked firmly under my arm. If I am lucky I may get a halfpenny for bringing back the paper and will be able to return to the shop where I will be able to buy three caramel sweets. They will last me a long while.

As I approach the top of the hill leading home, I meet the banister-scratching girl's older brother. He is with another boy and this gives him courage. He grabs me by the arm and says menacingly: 'You told on my sister, didn't you?'

I am terror stricken as I answer in a quivering voice: 'I ... I didn't.' He raises his hand to strike me, but somehow I twist away from his grasp and run as fast as I can, which really isn't very fast.

I am running for my life as a huge rock is sent tumbling down the hill after me. This is the reality of living in Limerick in the early 1960s. This is life and it is rough and tough.

It isn't long before the rock catches up with me. Well, it would have caught up with anyone, even an Olympic sprinter, never mind me. It hits me on the back of my bad left leg.

Enormous pain hits me. I ignore the pain and run on. Sheer terror now keeps me moving. As my left foot only lifts very slightly from the ground, the rock is like a terrier worrying my ankle, gashing it with his teeth. My poor leg is no match for it.

I can't escape the rock without leaving the footpath and running onto the road. Then, knowing my luck, I will probably be chased by a car. But as I round the corner, the rock, having no sense of direction, does not follow me. I stop running, I catch my breath and continue the rest of the way home, walking slowly, silently and grievously wounded.

When I arrive home, I hand my father the paper without a word. He offers me a halfpenny, but I do not take it. Halfpennies are scarce and one does not refuse them lightly. He does not accuse me of being moody. He knows there is something wrong and he asks, 'What's the matter, love?'

This show of concern for me is something I welcome. Everyone else would assume that I am just in a mood. But not Dad. He is different. He knows there is something wrong.

And with those caring words of his, I can no longer remain

silent. I become hysterical as I try to tell him what has happened. He lifts me onto his lap and very gently removes my shoe and my blood-stained sock. He looks at my heel, tiny, purple and oozing what little blood there is in that leg.

He is white with anger as he says to my mother: 'Mary, that boy is not going to get away with this.' With that my mother puts pen to paper, her answer to everything, and writes to the head nun, telling her what has happened to me because of the damage to the banister.

I will not take the note to school. It is Celia who takes it to the nun, who in turn reports the boy to the boys' school, where he is punished. But the matter is far from over.

Because I fear the schoolyard and being bullied going to and from school, I am always late back from lunch. That way I think I am safe. Only I haven't reckoned on boys mitching, or mooching as we called it. And, of course, with my luck I meet them, though as my rock thrower is with them, I think they might have been waiting for me.

This time rock thrower does not attack me himself. Instead he has his pal do it for him. It's like something out of the *Godfather* long before Marlon Brando stuffed his cheeks with cotton wool and began making offers no one could refuse.

'Is this the one, Don Corleone?' Luca Brazzi asks.

'Yeah. That's her.'

And then Lucca Brazzi proceeds to choke me. He places his hands tightly around my neck and squeezes, tighter and tighter until tears break from my eyes which surely must be bulging right out of their sockets. I begin to gag and because they are not the real Mafia, but mean, nasty cowards, they get frightened and let me go and run off.

But where do I go? Do I go home and complain again? If I do, the brutality will never stop. So do I continue onto school as if nothing's happened? I settle for the latter, never telling a soul about this murder attempt which has been made on me. But it is not the first secret I have kept and it will not be the last.

10

THE DOBBER CHAMPION

☙❧

So despite this attempt to murder me, and as if to make up for the terrible disappointment of failing as a ballerina, I make my stage debut at my very first Feile Luimni Concert. I am one of the four smallest children in the class and because of this we are put in the front row. Our class is reciting poetry. There are three benches on which we must stand: small girls in front; bigger girls behind us and the giants at the back.

My big worry isn't stage fright but how I am going to get up on the bench. I don't think it will look very professional if I put my hands on the bench to help myself get up on it. But I can't step up on it, left leg first, because the leg won't hold my weight. Neither can I place it on the ground and lead with my right leg. Same problem applies. I just hope no one wishes me luck by saying 'break a leg' because I just might do so.

I needn't have worried though because we get into our positions behind the curtain and I am able to get onto the bench with a helping hand – my own to be exact. But now, all during *The Battle of Fontenoy*, I worry about how I am going to get down gracefully.

The Battle of Fontenoy ends without casualties. But there is no relief for me and I watch helplessly as the curtain remains open and each girl gets gracefully down from the bench. As I agonise over what I should do, fate intervenes and takes the decision out of my hands. As the last girl gets down from my bench it begins to wobble. Self-preservation takes over, and I jump for dear life. But my heel gets caught and the bench topples over with a loud crash.

I blush with embarrassment, but console myself with the thought that at least I won't be shot. It isn't as if I'd deserted the battlefield in the midst of the action. So I compose myself and go backstage, glad that the ordeal is over. Well, the battle is over but there is one sniper in a gymslip waiting for me. 'It was you who knocked over the bench, wasn't it?' she says scornfully, taking away what little self-confidence I possessed. Should I have wanted to be an actress, destiny in a gymslip has decided for me at this moment that I shan't succeed. Stage fright takes on a new and terrible meaning. It now means not failing on the stage, but falling off it.

With my stage career at a premature end, I revert from culture back to nature. This is nature in the raw, where only the strongest and fittest survive. I am not very strong and I am not very fit. But I am brainy. Yet when all the girls form a gang, only the strongest and fittest girls are allowed to join. That means everyone, except me. And if I can't get into the gang I'll be all alone. So what am I to do? I approach the leader and ask: 'What have I to do to get into the gang?'

'Let's see,' she says, and I can see her thinking up an impossible test. 'Right,' she then says, a smirk of triumph on her face. 'You have to jump off the Hockey Wall.'

'What!' I exclaim in horror.

'We all did it,' she says, lying through her teeth. 'So if you want to be in the gang you'll have to do it too.'

'The Hockey Wall! But that's as high as Nelson's Pillar.' I knew he'd been up there at least 100 years and he hadn't jumped yet, despite the fact that he had two good legs and could hardly see how far down it was with his one eye.

'That's why you have to jump off it,' she sneered. 'That's the test.'

What can I do? I'll die if I have no one to play with. So I may as well die jumping off the Hockey Wall. 'I'll have to really think about it,' I say.

'OK. You've got three seconds. One, two, three. Right, what's your answer? Yes or no.'

'Yes. Having really thought about it, I'll do it.'

My friends stare at me in disbelief and awe. It must have been the self-same disbelief the sailors displayed on the Victory when Nelson said, 'Kiss me Hardy'. But do I also see great admiration there or is it maliciousness? I settle for admiration.

The word gets round. Joan is going to do the jump. Goody good, fraidy cat, who never does anything, is going to jump down off the Hockey Wall. There is more excitement than if I had been Evel Knievel about to jump the Grand Canyon. He may jump the canyon but he could never jump the Hockey Wall, not even on a motorbike.

The day dawns. There isn't much television coverage of historical events these days, otherwise both Terry Wogan and Gay Byrne would be here to televise this historic occasion. Feeling like a great hero, I climb up onto the great wall and then crawl petrified to the spot from where I am to jump.

Now I realise this is no ordinary jump. The wall which encloses the paupers' graveyard, and whose name is a mystery, is not only higher than Nelson's Pillar, but has bushes growing alongside it. So I will have to jump up over the bushes before I even begin my descent. I stand on the great height and for once look down on all my friends. It is a long, long way down.

'Jump,' they shout. But I can't. Standing on this great height and looking down on everyone, thoughts begin to pass through my mind. 'What if I break my good leg? I'll be murdered when I get home.'

'Jump,' they shout again.

'OK. In a minute,' I say.

My mind is in turmoil. If I don't jump I will never get in the gang. And more to the point, if I don't jump, how will I get down off the wall? Will it be easier to jump than to climb down? Oh, what can I do? As these thoughts filter through my brain, I know I must find courage somewhere.

'Are you going to jump or not?' My friends are growing impatient.

'OK. OK. In a minute. I have to think how to do it.'

'You just jump,' they say.

I start to think again. My friends don't like thinkers, or else they get tired of me thinking. Whichever it is, they decide to clear off and leave me alone on my pedestal. But if I want to be on a pedestal in their minds, I will have to jump. As I see them leaving I begin to think of Nelson again. He is going to remain a hero while it looks as if I will end up a coward. But if the latter thoughts induce a wish to jump, it is the fact that my friends are now shouting that the farmer is coming waving a big stick that ultimately spurs me to actually jump.

As I hit the ground my good leg buckles beneath me and my knee strikes me on the chin with a power that Cassius Clay would have been envious of. I lie sprawled on the ground, a hero. My friends run back and ask anxiously: 'Are you all right?'

I sit up and lie, just a bit. 'Of course I am. Nothing to it.' They are all in awe of me. Never before have they seen such bravery. I am their new hero. The word goes round that I've jumped off the Hockey Wall. But one of the gang wasn't present. 'Well, I didn't see her do it,' she says. 'So she'll have to do it again.'

Oh no. I am beginning to dislike pedestals. Which is just as well for I am about to be knocked off my pedestal once and for all – not by a doubting gang member, or by fear of heights, but by a simple pair of knitting needles.

Though now a fully-fledged gang member, I still don't know what membership entails – unless it means I can jump off walls, which doesn't seem of great value to me. What it certainly doesn't do is help me with my knitting, which we've just begun to learn at school. And despite being a gang member, I desperately want to be able to knit well.

An elderly neighbour woman always looked so peaceful and content sitting in the corner knitting, while her husband sat opposite her chewing tobacco and spitting in the fire. They certainly needed no Valium to help them through the twilight of their lives.

But now I need the Valium while learning to knit. And I so want to be able to master this lovely craft so I can knit a pair of red Teddy boy socks like those worn by Elvis Presley, and which look great on television, even in black and white.

My mother is a great knitter and she will knit a pair of socks for us children in a single night. There is always a bag of wool hanging on the back of the bedroom door. This wool comes from jumpers and cardigans that are beyond repair and which have been ripped out.

My mother rips out the old clothes while we hold the wool in our outstretched hands so that she can re-wind it. Because there are all sorts of different colours, she is able to knit the most beautiful Fairisle jumpers and cardigans.

She also saves the buttons which can be re-used. There is a blue canister of buttons on the dresser – all types of beautiful buttons – so we can end up with a variety of buttons on our cardigans.

When it comes to knitting though, I am not at all like my mother. I try and try but it is no use. I can start out with a mere twenty stitches and end up with 40. On four needles I am ten times worse. Yet at school I somehow manage to get away for a whole year without even finishing one sock.

Everyone else seems to be doing well on the four steel needles until they come to the square and the turning of the heel. For the life of me, I cannot grasp what needs to be done to succeed here. Many of the other girls also find this difficult, even the ones who are good at knitting and sewing.

So I think, quite logically, that if they find it difficult, I'll find it impossible. As each girl goes up to the teacher with her square and comes back down propelled on her way with a good thump on the back, I realise I can't risk venturing up there. And so each time I get to the square, I rip it back. And thus I continue all through the year. It's amazing how I ever get away with it. But it has one advantage. I do become quite proficient at ripping out. There are to be no knitted Teddy boy socks for me. I wonder now why I didn't ask my mother to knit them for me. Maybe I did and she didn't like Elvis.

Despite my failure at knitting, I am still determined that I am going to be a great housewife. So undeterred by my numerous failures in the field of housewifery, I begin my cooking career. And despite all the ridiculous things which happen because I take things literally, my parents still regard me as very sensible. If they tell me to do something, I do it exactly as instructed. Many's the time I am left in charge of the house, even though I am not the eldest. But maybe it's because I'm always determined to carry out my duties exactly to the letter.

Every evening after tea, I go outside to play. One evening, the children are playing a game which they call 'dobbers' and which is known as 'marbles' by the posh people who don't live in the back streets. I beg to be allowed to play and after one game I am obsessed and smitten, though initially I keep losing.

But then something extraordinary happens. I lose yet another game and have no dobbers left. The winner, as is the custom, gives me back a stake and a luck, which consists of two dobbers.

Now with my stake and a luck, I start winning. I win that evening and the next evening and the one after that. There is no stopping me. I have found my forte in life and soon I become a little tycoon. I own so many dobbers that I am in a position to sell them at six for a penny compared to the four for a penny which is charged in the shop. And no sooner have I sold them, than I win them back. The shy introvert has become aggressive and now I am universally feared once I have a dobber in my hand.

Soon I am unbeatable – a champion. My collection of dobbers stands at nearly 300 – big ones, small ones, lovely coloured ones, and china ones. I also have 'lead leads' which are ball bearings. The bigger ones are heavy and can send a glass dobber flying on its way. With the 'lead leads' it's so much easier to win, though I don't use them too often. I don't need to. I can win with any sort of dobber.

My collection is my pride and joy, and each evening, like Silas Marner with his gold, I take them out and count them. They are a symbol of wealth and of success, but all this has not been easily won. The secret of my success is dedication to my craft. I will play with anyone who calls, no matter what the weather. At times I feel pity for my opponents, having just sold them the dobbers I am in the process of winning back.

Eventually, I tire of my success because winning has become so easy. It is no longer a challenge and in the end I give all my dobbers away, not even bothering to charge for them. I decide that I'm not cut out to be a tycoon.

There are other attractions other than dobbers, one of which is water. And I am drawn to it as much as anyone else. But for me, just as for Napoleon long ago, it nearly becomes my Waterloo.

My Waterloo is a place not far from us called. 'The Swalley Hole' It is quite near the dump and is alleged to be capable of swallowing up anyone who falls in.

One day I find myself sitting on the walled edge of the hole along with my friend, a roller skate on one leg, and a cap bomber in my hand. We ponder the stories of this place and wonder if it is really capable of swallowing one up. We reach no conclusion and as if in frustration, I throw the bomber cap hard against the opposite wall. But as well as a loud bang, there is also the sound of a splash as the roller skate rolls down the side of the wall, pulling me with it into the hole. And now I find that the stories about this place are true, for it seems to be trying to pull me down into the dark depths.

My friend runs off calling wildly for help to our other friends who are searching for treasures in the dump. All the while I can feel myself being pulled down. 'Come back,' I scream, desperately holding onto the edge of the wall while the weight of the roller skate threatens to dislodge me. I know if I let go my tenuous grip, I will sink down to the bowels of the earth and never be found again.

I hope that there are no treasures to be found in the dump today because then my friends will surely not come back to rescue me. I will be forgotten in the excitement of the find. But eventually my friend returns with reinforcements and finds me, waist deep in the water and clinging desperately to the side of the wall.

They pull me out, soaked to the skin and trembling in terror. The hole has been denied its right this time. But it can wait, silent and dark and always ready. There will be other children and other opportunities. It will bide its time.

I learn a very valuable lesson this day. It is that one's hold on life is no stronger than a thread. At any moment it can snap, even under so little a weight as a single roller skate. And so you must grasp life with both hands while you can. But I will learn too that that isn't always so easy, because there are always people and fate willing to snatch that life from your grasp and dash it to pieces before your very eyes.

11

LADY OF THE DANCE

❦

By 1963 the 'swinging sixties' are well under way but I am too young yet for swinging. In fact, I am still trying to learn how to knit, never mind swing. And despite the fact that I've failed miserably at knitting a sock, I now have the momentous task of knitting a jumper which will be worn on the last day of the school year.

I am so proud when I master a lovely stitch that my mother has taught me – no common plain and purl for the master – me. So I begin and miracle of miracles, I don't appear to be having any problem with the two needles. The back and front of the jumper turn out just fine. It is the sleeves that turn out to be my downfall.

My mother tells me that I need to increase the stitches for the sleeves as I go along so as to get the tapered shape right. And I follow this instruction to the letter. I increase and increase and increase until the sleeve is as wide as the back and front put together.

Despite being brainy, I realise too late that something is wrong and I go to my mother for help. Now she puts me right when it's too late. She tells me that at some point I should have stopped increasing. When I'm knitting the second sleeve I should come to her and she will advise me.

I don't really have time to alter the first sleeve so I cast it off and begin the second one. With advice from my mother, it turns out all right. So the jumper is now sewn up. It looks very pretty, but boy is it uncomfortable. And it's just my luck that the only time that I've had a brand new jumper to wear, I feel terrible in it. Not only that, but now I will have to wear it until it wears out.

On the last day at school before the holidays, I stand in my beautiful pink jumper and try and hide a huge excess of knitting under one arm. Now I know why Napoleon always had his hand stuck inside his jacket. He was trying valiantly to hide an excess of sleeve.

Anyway, I am not wearing that jumper some weeks later when I pay my regular visit to the Orthopaedic Clinic. A new surgeon has taken over there and he wants to operate on me. He can't wait to get at me with the knife. He is very very keen indeed, but my mother is more cautious. 'What will the operation do for her?' she asks him.

'If it's successful, she'll be able to walk perfectly,' he replies.

'And if not?' my mother asks.

'Then,' he says, 'she could end up in a wheelchair.'

As there is no six-month guarantee being offered, my mother refuses to allow me to undergo the surgery. 'But you can't have her going around like that for the rest of her life,' he protests. I reckon he doesn't like people with limps. Anyway, my mother refuses to budge and it seems as if I'll have to go around 'like that' for the rest of my life.

'Well, if you won't consent to an operation,' he adds, with injured pride, 'there is nothing more I can do for her.'

Faced with this ultimatum from a person in high authority whom she has learned must always be obeyed, my mother weakens and decides to seek the advice of the other doctor who is present. 'I'd leave very well alone,' he says, and she agrees to accept his opinion which corresponds with her own. I will continue to come for check-ups, but this, it now appears, is as good as I am going to get.

As we are about to leave, my mother suddenly asks, 'What about the spud water? Will I continue with that?'

'What spud water?' The surgeon is obviously astonished.

'I've been bathing her leg in it for years,' my mother tells him. 'It's supposed to be a great cure for the bad leg.' She seems to fail to see the problem with this remark. My leg is as bad, or as good, as it's ever been, spud water or not.

'Oh forget that nonsense,' he says dismissively.

Now that I'm finished with the hospital and the possibility of further operations, I decide that I will never wear the big boot again. I only wore it when going for the check ups anyway in case the unfortunate doctors would think that they hadn't cured me. And I also make the momentous decision that from now on I'm not going to stand for the spud water either. Instead I set my sights on being the Queen of Irish dancing, despite my failure to be a prima ballerina.

All my friends are having Irish dancing lessons and I want to learn too. I pester my mother until she agrees that I can go. I don't know where she gets the necessary ninepence from, but somehow she gets it and off I go. No sooner do I get to the hall than I regret having given up wearing my big boot, for the teacher is wearing two big boots similar to mine, and with them she pounds on the floor. Despite obviously having polio in both legs, she seems to enjoy this show of aggression.

The first lesson begins with a line of children whom she calls 'the beginners'. I am one of them. 'Right children,' she says. 'Stand straight and do exactly as I do. Now, left foot back. Right foot forward. And one two three four five six seven.' She pounds the floor and we all copy her. 'Left foot, one two three. Right foot, one two three.' There is no music but that is more than made up for by the rousing beat of the feet. I am elated. I can dance. I will be a great dancer.

There and then I have a vision. I see the future. It's 1994 and I'm dancing with a man in a dark billowing shirt and funny hair, who's making as much racket as a troop of elephants wearing big boots on their four feet. 'Hi, Jean,' he says to me. 'How do you like this new dance I've invented?'

'It's Joan,' I say, peeved that he's got my name wrong. 'And I thought you were Rudolph Nureyev!'

Ah, dreams. They make me practise all week and I can hardly wait for the next lesson. Soon I will be able to dance a jig or a reel in soft shoes, and then I'll get to dance the hornpipe in the hard soled shoes. The' Siege of Ennis' and the 'Walls of Limerick' are just waiting for me. Cromwell couldn't knock down the walls, but I will. Limerick, Ireland, the world – they are just waiting for me.

And then I have lesson two a week later. It's another nine pence and again my mother produces a miracle. First off, we repeat what we learned the previous week and then begin the new lesson. It's so exciting, I can't wait. I keep wishing the teacher would hurry up

'Right then,' she says eventually. 'We'll move on to the next part. Now, right foot hop, two three four five six seven.' So far so good. Then it's 'left foot hop, two, three, hop, two three.' Left foot can hear but left foot can't hop. Left foot will not hop. I try and try until I fall in a heap on the floor. 'You can't do it,' she says. 'Stand out of the line.' I creep away to a corner, shamed and humiliated. Talk about getting your ninepence worth!

But I am determined to persevere. If the teacher can hop so well with polio in both feet, I think, then I should certainly be able to do so with polio in one foot. Over the following days I spend hours and hours trying to learn to hop on the left foot, but to no avail. I lift the leg up and down with my hands, I swing it about. But as soon as it's left to its own devices, it won't do anything, never mind hop.

I have been told, or learned, that the brain is responsible for all our movements, that it sends the messages to each limb to move. It does this automatically without being asked or told, or so I am led to believe. So I order my brain to send a message to my left foot to hop. But it appears not to be listening. In the end I have to concede that my second great dancing career is over and a very precious 1/6 wasted into the bargain.

While no one remembers the day my career ended, everyone remembers where they were on that fateful night in November when President Kennedy is shot. I'm no exception to this general rule. I am watching TV in my friend Theresa's house. We still don't possess a television. In fact, we cannot afford anything other than the very basics.

So in order to see some television I have oftentimes to beg. It's fine if myself and Theresa are best friends – then I can call into her house any time. But when we fall out, there is no television for me.

Sometimes in this situation, her mother will let me in to watch television, much to the annoyance of Theresa. And so it's many's the night I spend under their kitchen table watching *The Fugitive, Batt Masterson, Palladin* and *The Thin Man*.

On this dark November evening we are watching *The Thin Man*. The girl in the picture is tied up and struggling to free herself. The camera pans to the door, the knob turns slowly. Under the table, I am riveted to the screen.

And then we have a newsflash. President Kennedy has been shot in Dallas. I am only twelve years old, but even at this tender age I can understand and sense the awfulness of it. I know something terrible has happened.

I am aware of the joy his visit to Ireland in the summer brought to the people of the country. When he came to Limerick, Mrs Fitz herself got to shake his hand and she told me she would not wash her hand for days afterwards. Most of the houses I know have pictures of John F. Kennedy and the pope on their walls. We just have the pope. We cannot afford JFK yet.

I run home with the news, heartbroken about the shooting. But weeks later I've all but forgotten it. Now all I'm wondering about is what happened to the girl in *The Thin Man*.

I am twelve years of age and I'm growing up, and I want to have great adventures like the girl in *The Thin Man*. I want to go out into the great big world. But not too far to begin with. So I take my first step by venturing into the city for the first time on my own.

I feel like a real grown up as I get on the bus on my own and make my way into town. I feel very independent and I know my mother will be proud of me. I have a number of shops to visit. I go to E.G. Fitzes, where they sell the cheapest bacon and then to Winstons where I can get the Green Shield Stamps. With these, one day we will be able to get a companion set for beside the fire, a log basket, and all the other little luxuries that we cannot afford.

I am delighted with myself when I complete the shopping and am ready for the return journey home. With my bags of heavy shopping, I wait for the bus. I am tired and I'm looking forward to a sit down.

At last the bus arrives, but there are no vacant seats available and so I have to stand, my bags of shopping a hindrance in the narrow isle. Being small, I cannot reach the overhead grab bars, and I am left to the mercy of the G Forces.

But the G Forces have no mercy and further more, do not keep me pinned in any shape or form. Having no balance, as the bus starts, the G forces also start and throw me onto the floor. When I manage to get up my face is bright red.

Some minutes later the bus stops and I go down again. And so begins my most unusual journey. Each time the bus starts or stops I go down. By the time I eventually get a seat I have got used to getting up, because there are a lot of stops between the town and Killeely. Yet despite this constant falling down, I never let go of the bags of shopping. By the time I get home, I'm beginning to wonder about the wisdom of venturing into the big world.

12

WISDOM AND UNDERSTANDING

❦

By 1964 the swinging sixties are really under way. Elvis Presley is all the rage and the Beatles are about to take the world by storm. I am still too young to go dancing, but my youth cannot prevent me listening to this great rock 'n' roll music – 'The Hippy Hippy Shakes', '5,4,3,2,1', 'Don't Throw Your Love Away' – and Elvis Presley, always Elvis. I can never tire of 'Wooden Heart'. But I am about to learn that there is another meaning to rock and roll. It's a much more dangerous meaning – worse than the imaginary fears of the older generation who can only shake their heads in despair at the youth of today.

I am a coward. Or so all my brave friends keep telling me. But I believe that coward is just another word for sensible, and that they are the ones who are stupid. Sensible children have no friends. So I find I have to be stupid in one way in order to be sensible in another.

The bread van comes daily to deliver the bread to the local shops. A popular adventure for my friends is to crouch behind the bread van when it stops outside a shop. Then, as soon as the driver climbs back into the cab, they clamber up on the rear bumper and hold on for dear life to the door handle. When the van drives off, they get a great spin. Cars are rare in these days and any kind of free jaunt is a great treat.

But being a sensible coward, I refuse to take part in this foolishness. 'OK,' my friends say. 'If you're going to be a coward, then you can't play with us.' So much for jumping off the Hockey Wall, I think. But as not being allowed to play is a fate worse than dying while jumping off a wall, I am shamed into being a great hero.

The day dawns. The bread van arrives in the road. I hide behind it with my friends and climb onto the bumper along with them when the van moves off. We hold on tightly to the door handle and as we gather speed slowly, it feels exhilarating. What had I been afraid of, I ask myself? One must live; one must enjoy life; one must go places even if only holding onto bread van door handles. But I am about to learn that I had been right all along to be both cautious and afraid.

My experienced companions know at what point to jump off. I don't. And as I ponder this vital question, they abandon ship. One by one they leap off, leaving me alone and hanging on for dear life.

Meanwhile, the van is picking up speed. It's travelling faster and faster. Invisible forces seem to be trying to drag me off my perilous perch. I realise that if I don't get off soon, I'll be taken right into the city. Then I'll have to walk home. Now that would be really stupid – to take a ride for fun and have to walk back.

By now my 'dear' friends are running after the van and shouting at me to get off. 'How?' I scream.

'Let go of the handle and jump,' they shout.

Of course, I trust them. I let go of the handle and try to jump backwards. Now it is hard enough for me to jump forwards, never mind try out such a complex manoeuvre. So as I let go of the handle, I fall onto the road and roll forward. When I come to a stop, I lie sprawled and injured. As the van continues on its way, the driver oblivious to the load he has just lost, I rock myself to and fro to try and alleviate the pain which seems to occupy every square inch of my poor body.

So much for being a hero. It isn't that easy after all, being brave. I've learned that lesson at least. As I pick myself up, I learn too that it is my pride that is most injured and I promise myself that I won't go rocking and rolling again in a hurry. Not unless there's a smooth wooden dance floor without wheels, a gorgeous Teddy boy with his comb in his back pocket, his quiff, and his hair at the back in a ducktail. Yet that is a long way off yet. I am still too young, too inquisitive, too gullible, too imaginative and too timid to be let loose on an unsuspecting public.

But before I can even get started, I am to be sent to rehab. And I don't even know who's responsible for this. Rehab, I know, is where the criminals go when they are released from prison – only I haven't even gone to prison yet. I'm not a criminal. Well, OK, I did jump on the bread van, but I was the only one who got hurt then. Yet I am the one who's going to rehab, to be rehabilitated I assume. I don't know what they intend to do with me and I never really find out, because on the day my mother takes me there, they're closed and we never do go back again. So I never really get rehabilitated, which probably explains a great deal.

It's not rehabilitating I need. In many ways I am much too quiet. I never want to fight – well, I'm fully aware that physically I'm not able to fight. It isn't that I'm not strong enough. It is due to the fact that I have no balance. So no matter how I'm hit, hard or not, I just fall over. With even a slight push, I will go down quicker than a boxer who's being paid, or threatened, to throw a fight. But all that will soon change.

I am about to make my confirmation. Once confirmed, I will become both brave and strong. Or so I'm led to believe. Once I get strong, I'll be able to fight everyone without falling down at all.

Before this, I have to get all the clothes for the big day. But once again, this is a major problem. My mother cannot afford to buy them. There is a scheme available where you can get a 'docket' for £3.00 at the local shop. We apply for the docket and each day I have to go along to the shop to see if the docket is ready. Even at my age, I find this humiliating and dread it.

After a great many visits, the magic 'docket' appears. But by now I've been so humiliated that the 'docket' is all but detestable to me. And it isn't even charity. It has to paid back at perhaps a shilling a week with a very high rate of interest added on.

Only certain shops will accept the docket, so we are limited as to choice. We go to Roches Stores, 'the caring store', and there my mother picks out a cotton dress. Most of the other girls will have beautiful nylon dresses in pinks and blues and yellows. I will have to make do with this staid cotton one.

The shop assistants who are dealing with us ask my mother if we need a cardigan because the dress only has short sleeves. 'Ah no,' my mother says. 'I couldn't afford a cardigan as well.' The assistants go into a huddle and we wait.

As the dress is being wrapped up, a white cardigan in a plastic wrapper is placed beside it. My mother repeats that she cannot afford the cardigan. 'It's alright, missus,' one of the assistants say. 'We've bought that between us.' It is a simple, kind gesture which I do not fully appreciate. Yet I will never forget that kindness.

I will need a coat too, and this is purchased in another store where they sell cheap coats for tall people who are not making their confirmation. The coat reaches my ankles, even though the present style is worn to the knees. Poor people always buy clothes that are too big for them so they can grow into them. I feel a right idiot in the long coat. But it will have to last for years. And it will be serviceable for even longer than it would be for a normal child because it takes poor children a long time to grow due to poor nutrition.

And so the day dawns. I am to be confirmed in my cotton dress, white cardigan, long coat and black patent shoes. I am about to become stronger and wiser at last. We have to choose a new name for this ceremony and I choose Bernadette, after my favourite saint. She had it tough too.

After the anointing with Chrism, the Bishop slaps each candidate on the cheek. This is supposed to be a symbol of the strength one is about to become endowed with. But his hand appears to slip when it is my turn and I get a fair old whack. I don't worry about this. I know it's for that extra bit of strength that I am going to need for the future.

Now, I think, I'm ready to take on the whole world. So after-wards, when I think no one is looking, I flex my muscles to see if there is any improvement. I'm convinced there is, which says a great deal for the wisdom and understanding I was supposed to get too. But when I do become sensible, if not exactly wise, it becomes apparent that it is not physical strength that is required for survival but the gift of inner strength, and I am going to need a great deal of that.

While I'm supposed to be getting strength and wisdom and all that sort of thing, the great world itself spins merrily away in space. And all around the world, a great many odd things are happening. For a start, a Berlin Wall is built and we hear of peo-ple being shot almost every day trying to cross it. It is a great mys-tery to me why it's needed at all and why people want to escape from behind it. Maybe they want to see what's on the other side and I wonder why they don't put a few windows or holes in it and then people could look out.

But even stranger than the Berlin Wall is the fact that someone has hung an Iron Curtain somewhere in Europe. There's a lot of discussion on the radio about this Iron Curtain and the things that are going on behind it. I am intrigued by this because even a child couldn't hide behind our curtains, they are so short and scanty. But this Iron Curtain is really extraordinary. According to the radio reports, there are millions of people behind it. Puzzled by this, I ask my Dad about it. As I know from previous experience, he knows everything. 'What else is behind this Iron Curtain?' I ask him, 'apart from all those millions of people?'

'Eastern Europe, love,' he says

'Eastern Europe!' It must be a very big curtain indeed, I think. 'But why is it there?' I ask.

'To stop people crossing over from one side to the other.'

'Why?'

'Well Europe was divided after the war and the Iron Curtain separates Eastern Europe from Western Europe.'

But that still doesn't tell me what the Iron Curtain looks like.

Now I want to see it for myself and find the answers to all the questions whirling about in my head. Like what material is it made of? Is it really made of iron? Who takes it down and washes it? How big is it? Could a child creep under it? What does it hang on, tracks or poles (I suppose it's hung on really heavy steel poles?) Was it ever drawn, and if so, who was strong enough to draw it?

But these questions are not to be answered. And when they are, the answers turn out to be bizarre. It seems that the Iron Curtain is actually invisible. So I decide it must have been made by the same people who made the emperor's clothes.

I could have made clothes for the emperor and they would have been magnificent – as magnificent as only a great creative mind like mine could dream up. But as for the actual making itself – the cutting out and the sewing – well, that would be a different matter. My hands were not meant for such things.

This is a fact I come to realise at the beginning of the new school term when we have to learn dressmaking. Many's the time I find myself wishing that I was making clothes for the emperor. At least that way, no one would have to see my poor efforts. But it is a forlorn wish, for as far as I know, emperors didn't wear slips, the garment I am trying to make. Slips are what most girls wore under their dresses in the olden days before Levi Strauss stopped playing 'The Blue Danube' on his fiddle, riveted some old canvas together, and came up with 'blue jeans'.

Anyway, whatever about Levi Strauss and his designer denims, I have to make a slip. But before I can begin, I have to purchase the material. My mother advises me to go to Denis Moran's shop in the city centre where material can be bought cheaply. I go to the shop and, not seeing any material, I find myself at the counter. It is very high and I place my fingers on the edge and pull myself up so that I can look over it.

There is one man beside me, presumably not there to buy material for a slip, and a number of other men behind the counter. They don't appear to have any notion of serving me. But that doesn't prevent them from staring at me in a bemused way. 'Typical,' I think, feeling annoyed at being ignored. 'There are enough men here to serve a shop full of customers, and they won't bother serving me, even though it is obvious I am hanging on for dear life.'

Eventually the man beside me asks me what do I want and I think, 'It's a bit much when a customer starts asking me what I want.' I ignore him. Instead, I look around and notice a lot of stacked boxes on the shelves behind me. Only then do I realise that I am inside the counter and that the 'customer' is in fact the sales assistant. No wonder the real customers, outside the counter, are bemused.

I am mortified. And when I tell the man that I am looking for material to make a slip, I am doubly mortified when he informs me that I am in their 'man's shop'. The one I want is a little up the street.

I eventually get the material and manage to make what I think is a pretty good slip. Even if it doesn't live up to its name and slip on and off easily, it certainly feels secure and I am proud of my year's work. But the teacher is horrified and says that no self-respecting girl would wear such an ill-fitting garment. Just as well Levi Strauss didn't have her as a teacher. If he had, he might have stuck with the fiddle and just been famous for a few old dance tunes.

13

THE BIRDS AND THE BEES

☙☙

It only seems like yesterday since I joined the 'babies' and now it's my last term at National School. And having spent eight years on my education, I pride myself on knowing everything. So it isn't unusual for other girls in my class to come to me for help with any problem that's proving difficult.

Normally we only have our English books at school for reading, and one soon gets fed up reading about holidays by the sea, especially when we have never seen the sea. And all those great adventures picking blackberries and making jam and playing snap apple on Halloween night, don't exactly set the pulse racing. We couldn't afford the sugar for the jam and anyway, what would we drink our tea out of if we actually filled all those jam jars with jam?

So naturally there is great excitement among us when a set of encyclopaedias appear at school. These large books fascinate us girls. Most are particularly curious about the volume which contains the letter B, especially the entry for Baby.

It's always in demand and they quarrel continuously about who should have it first. But I don't bother. Not me. Big deal, I think. Who wants to know about babies?

Anyway, I have more interesting entries to read, like those for Neanderthal Man, Peking Man and Homo Sapiens. But there is obviously some fascination in that other volume because the pages are dog eared in comparison to the rest of the book. A great many pupils have left evidence of their unbridled curiosity behind them.

One day, I am deep in thought about my origins and the origins of my Neanderthal cousins, when some of the girls look up from the dog-eared pages and ask me if I know the facts of life. What a silly question. Of course I know the facts of life. I know the facts of everything.

'I do,' I reply, proud, as usual, that my immense knowledge is being sought. 'But I can't remember them right now.'

They dare to laugh at me and I become annoyed with myself that I can't remember them all right now. I try to save face. 'There are four altogether,' I pronounce with absolute conviction. 'But I just can't think of any of them at the moment.'

They snigger at this and I realise that they must think me a right fool. Before I can retort, they put another question to me. 'So do you know where babies come from, then?' they ask, sniggering uncontrollably now.

I realise they are making fun of me. But I don't even bother answering them. I know they expect me to say that the stork brings them down from heaven in a basket, hidden beneath a head of cabbage. But at fourteen, I'm well aware that this isn't so. I now know for certain that a nurse, or a doctor if you're important enough, gets them from under a head of cabbage in the vegetable garden out at the Regional Maternity Hospital.

When they stop tormenting me and return to reading about babies, I rack my brains trying to think of the facts of life. But I just can't remember them at all. It's just as well, for I'm sure what I would come up with would confirm for them that I am a right fool indeed.

Anyway, after a while I give up pondering the facts of life and return to what's really puzzling me. This is the vexed question of beneath what vegetable Neanderthal man (while he was still in nappies, of course) was found. I do know that they didn't have Neanderthal heads of cabbage in those days and they certainly didn't have a Regional Maternity Hospital. But when I leave the National School for good that summer, the question remains unanswered and I feel a failure.

***

L eaving the National School is a watershed. I am now sup-posed to be grown up but my body seems unaware of this fact and steadfastly refuses to soar upwards. My sister Celia has a similar growth problem which she tries to combat by drinking Fry's cocoa every night. It has a picture of a very happy family on the yellow packet and has a caption which declares: Growing up on Fry's.

But I don't like cocoa and so I seem doomed to my fate. While Celia drinks gallons of cocoa and remains small, I drink none and remain small. The only difference between us is that she is actual-ly taller than me, but I look taller. I only looked at the box and I think that seems to have worked out much better.

We are becoming teenagers and now my mother tries to impress on us the facts of life – the elusive facts which had so humiliated me. But she tries to impart this knowledge without really telling us anything – quite a feat indeed.

We have always been brought up to be very modest and decent which seems to have entailed not showing our knickers to anyone, especially while still wearing them. As I am mortified that anyone should see them, I fail to see why I'm being admon-ished to keep them hidden when I spend most of my time trying to ensure that no one sees them anyway.

But now my mother seems to emphasise this more and more. 'And the fact of life,' she says, 'is that you must never ever go nowhere alone with a man.' Knowledge at last! Here was one of those elusive facts. And here too was my chance.

'What are the other three, Mam?' I ask.

'Three what?' She is puzzled.

'The three facts.'

'Just do as I tell you,' she says a bit abrupt. 'Then you won't need to know them. Just make sure you don't be alone with a man morning, noon or night.'

'But why?' I ask.

'Because I'm telling you. That's why.'

And that was that. So I decide to consult my sister Kathleen on the matter. 'Mam is right,' she tells me. 'You should never be alone with a man because they're always looking for it.'

'Looking for what?' I ask.

'Never mind,' she says, blushing, and refuses to say any more. So I'm pretty much left in the dark on this matter.

Then a few days later my mother's advice is put to the test. I am alone in the house when a young local fellow calls to the door. He tells me that he has some electrical job to do in the house.

'Well you can't come in,' I say.

'Why not?'

'Because it's morning. That's why.'

'What's that got to do with it?'

'I can't say.'

'Look,' he says. 'Your mother asked me to check some electric wires under the floorboards in one of the upstairs bedrooms.' (A likely story!) 'Now can I come in or not?'

'Well, there's no one here,' I say.

'You're here,' he says

'Well, you don't think that I'm going upstairs alone with you, do you?' I say.

He must know the same fact of life I know because he goes very red in the face and after telling me to tell my mother he called, he goes away. I am very proud of myself for having avoided being alone with a man, especially as it was the morning, one of the times my mother had particularly pointed out when they were to be avoided. She had not said anything about the evening, but that made sense. I knew they'd be too tired if they were at 'it'''(whatever 'it' was) morning, noon and night.

When my mother eventually returns and I tell her I wouldn't

let the young man in, she gets annoyed with me. 'Why didn't you let him in?' she demands. 'I've been waiting weeks for him to call.'

'But you told me not to go anywhere alone with a man. Morning noon or night, you said. So I couldn't let him in, could I?' She casts her eyes to heaven, but she has no answer for me.

During the long summer holidays, there is more time for play and so much more opportunity for squabbling and fighting. But I am very timid. I will not stand up for myself and so I am miserable. Celia usually stands up for me, but I realise that I must learn to defend myself.

I confide my fears in Celia and ask her what I should do. She gives me great advice about how to react to a situation. 'You must never show them you're afraid,' she says.

'But what will I do if they say they'll hit me?' I ask.

'Tell them to do it. In fact, say, 'Go on, do it, do it, do it,' and they'll back off.'

'And what will I do if they do hit me?' I ask.

'Hit them back.'

What could be easier than that? So off I go – fearless at last. No one is going to meddle with me again.

It isn't long before the inevitable confrontation takes place, but I am ready. Boy, am I ready! The enemy, who is also a friend, begins by attacking me, verbally. But eventually it turns physical. 'Oh go away or I'll really hit you,' she says with contempt.

But I am not afraid any more. 'Go on.' I say 'Do it. Do it. Do it.' I raise my voice a little each time. And she does it! Thwack! Right across the face with her open hand. Well, that first bit of advice hasn't worked, I think. But I still have that second bit up my sleeve and I follow it to the letter. I hit her back. Yet she hits me again even harder and again I retaliate. However, while her blows are akin to those of a professional fighter, mine are just little tips and taps.

It's no use, I realise. I am not a fighter, at least not in the physical sense. I can feel the tears in my eyes. But I think, no! The enemy mustn't see me crying. And so I leave the arena a yellow coward. I go straight to my bedroom where I cry tears of humiliation, frustration and rage.

'What happened?' my sister asks when she comes and finds me.

'I won't listen to you again,' I cry. 'I had a fight with a friend, she hit me and I hit her back, and then she really hit me hard and it hurt and everyone saw it and I had to go away.'

'Well, it's better to have fought and lost than not to have fought at all,' she says.

'If you ask me,' I reply, 'it's even better to run away.'

'But you stood up to her anyway,' she says.

Yes, I had stood up to her. But I will never stand up to anyone again. I know now that it's far more humiliating to hit someone than to be hit by them. In one fell swoop, I've become a pacifist.

***

In September 1965 I begin my short career at secondary school, which is certainly new and different. Here, among all the other subjects, there is cookery to be learned. I love the smell of baking and the look of decorated cakes, and always longed to be able to cook. But like the knitting and sewing, it seems as if it isn't going to be that easy for me. Things seems to go wrong even before I get into the classroom.

First off, I fall while running for the bus. I have my ingredients for making scones – milk, eggs and flour – in my schoolbag and I hope they won't be all mixed before I even get to school. But when I do get there, I discover spilt milk, broken eggs and flour in the bag. The teacher takes one look and declares there will be no baking for me today!

When it comes to a test in pastry making, I hope to do much better, however. After all, I should be an expert in this field, having watched my father making the pastry for apple pies on numerous occasions. Mind you, he has never made jam tarts, which is the task facing me.

While the test is in progress, the teacher walks around the kitchen watching our efforts. I have my piece of dough rolled out neatly, and just to show off I pick it up without breaking it, turn it over, and begin rolling the other side.

'Failed,' she says, and walks on.

I am devastated. I haven't even cut out the pastry yet and there's still the jam to go in them, never mind taking into consideration the mammoth task of putting them in the oven and waiting for them to bake. All this to go, and she's failed me already.

What have I done wrong, I wonder, as I complete the procedure and wait for my tarts to bake. The only consolation is the happy knowledge that even if they burn, she can't fail me twice.

Later, I ask one of the other girls what I did wrong and discover the grave mistake I made. I should have picked up the pastry on the rolling pin. Imagine having failed over that! Whoever picks up pastry on a rolling pin? My father didn't even have a rolling pin and had to make do with a Guinness bottle for rolling out. And he certainly didn't pick up the pastry with the bottle either. But he did drink the contents as a pick-me-up for himself.

I feel terribly wronged. I am certain this set back is going to ruin my cooking career. Mind you the jam tarts are delicious and I eat most of them on the way home. Perhaps the teacher should have had one herself and she might have thought differently about my culinary skills.

One day, this same teacher tells us that it is vitally important to be back at school at exactly 2pm as we are going to make Genoa cake. This takes a half hour to mix, and one and a half hours to bake. So the time factor is very tight. But despite all the warnings, I still miss the bus and arrive half an hour late. By now all the Genoa cakes are about to go into the oven.

This has worked in my favour. I now have the sole attention of the teacher and eventually my cake too goes into the oven. But, of course, when the bell sounds, my cake still isn't baked. So the teacher has to stay back – poor thing.

By the time the summer holidays come around I'm sure the

poor teacher is looking forward to escaping from the cooking as much as I am. I'm sick of getting the ingredients and I've no doubt she's sick of seeing me make a disaster with them. But if she does escape, I don't. I am still sent to the Corner Shop for the messages on a daily basis.

One day I go to the shop as usual – only it isn't usual today. I can't breathe. When I arrive at the shop I lay my arms on the counter and try to speak, but no words come. I try again and eventually I manage to gasp, 'Half a stone of potatoes and a head of cabbage.'

The shopkeeper looks at me with concern. 'Look love, you're awfully sick. You'd better go home.' It seems I am very ill but I don't realise it until he tells me. And he should know. After all he is a grown up. Well, I will go home, once I get the shopping.

I get the potatoes and the largest head of cabbage I can find, then set off for home. What a long journey it turns out to be. As I walk, the potatoes and cabbage seem to get heavier and heavier. Once, I even stop and look under the head of cabbage to make sure there isn't a baby hidden underneath.

At the top of our street I glance down and it seems endless. I feel like the hero in the desert who sees a mirage in the far distance. Like him, I think I will never get there. But like John Wayne I keep going and going and get there eventually. And unlike those heroes, I don't fall and have to crawl the last few yards.

But maybe I should have done so, because then I might have got some sympathy (I would have to be dying to be taken to see a doctor). Instead I am told off for taking so long. Too breathless to react, I flop in a chair until I recover. For days afterwards I am frightened of this sickness returning and spoiling my summer. But it doesn't recur. However, it is only biding its time.

I love the summer especially because I can wear sandals – that is when I can find a suitable pair, for it is always a nightmare trying to get shoes to fit me. Sometimes a bit of light relief is needed to dispel my gloom.

One day I see Clarkes Shoes' boast in the window of one of

the more upmarket shops: 'Have your feet measured on our foot gauge and get shoes to fit you'. That'll do me, I think. So in I go.

'Does this measuring gadget really work?' I ask the assistant.

'Oh yes,' she enthuses. 'Everyone should really have their feet measured before they purchase a pair of shoes.'

'What if one foot is smaller?' I ask. I am being honest in a dishonest sort of way.

'Well, in most people there's a tendency for the left foot to be slightly smaller,' she says. 'But we can always supply the correct size shoes for each person.'

'So you should be able to supply me.' (I hope not, because I have no money).

'Yes. Of course.'

She has played right into my hands – or rather feet. 'OK,' I say. 'I'll try it.' I take off my right shoe and the foot is measured – a pretty normal, wide fitting. Now I take off the left shoe and the foot gauge takes a nose-dive, two and a half sizes down and a much narrower fitting.

'Is this foot gauge correct?' the astonished assistant asks a senior colleague. It seems it is. I assure her too that the gauge is correct, but as I'd already pointed out to her, my left leg is a smaller size than my right one. I also point out to her that she has promised me I will get the correct size shoes – except it turns out to be Mission Impossible! The look of horror and bewilderment on her face 'makes my day'. And 'Dirty Harry' is nowhere in sight.

14

POLES AND POEMS

☙❧

It is the summer of 1966 and the World Cup is being played in England. Soon I become bored with all the football on the television. I know nothing about football except that according to my Irish book the Irish for football is *cluice peile*.

However, during the tournament the name Pele keeps cropping up. He is referred to regularly as the greatest football player in the world. Now, this interests me. Why wouldn't it when the greatest player in the history of football should be called after the game in Irish? Well, at least the second bit. He must surely be our greatest honorary Irishman. (Jack Charlton is also playing in the tournament but at this time is only training to be an honorary Irishman!)

I am really amazed when I eventually see Pele. He has a raincoat draped over his shoulders and is limping along the edge of the pitch in a similar manner to myself. According to the commentator, he has been kicked out of the game, which I think is a pretty nasty thing to do to someone with a bad leg. I sympathise with him, though my brother tells me that Pele doesn't have polio.

Pele seems a funny colour even for an honorary Irishman. Maybe he only looks that colour because he's been kicked black and blue. I watch now in the hope that he will re-appear. But he doesn't and my brother informs me he's gone to Brazil. Who can blame him? If I'd been treated like him, I'd go to Brazil too.

While Pele may be the best footballer in the world, the one the girls are all crazy about this summer is Bobby Moore. I have to admit he is fabulous looking, but I can never understand why he always seems to be photographed beside a man with no teeth called Nobby, another with no hair called Bobby and yet another man who has two Christian names, Martin and Peter, but no surname.

As the World Cup ends with Bobby Moore hoisted onto the shoulders of the toothless and the hairless and the surnameless, I have my own problems to contend with. I am beginning to develop into a woman. I am!

I am becoming very aware of 'bumps'. They seem to be sprouting everywhere. It is very embarrassing. I think I am evolving too quickly. Charles Darwin had mentioned a figure of millions of years, but I could have told him that it happens much faster than that.

I also discover that I possess a major fault. My nose. My friends keep making remarks about it and I become very self-conscious. It does have a bump on it – the nose that is - but I am reliably informed that it is a knowledge bump. In my ignorance, I believe this. It never enters my head to wonder how, if it is a knowledge bump, I didn't know about it until someone told me.

I find myself so conscious of my numerous protuberences that whenever I am introduced to a fella, I try to hide them. So I fold my arms across my chest and cover my nose with my hand. This silly habit goes on until Celia informs me that I look better with the bump on my nose. And anyway, with the growing size of my chest, no fella in his right mind will ever notice my nose.

But it is the autumn of 1966 before I find my very own Bobby Moore in the guise of a boy who only thinks he can play football. I fall in love, a sign that I am growing up at last and that the hormones producing those bumps are having other effects on me as well.

I am playing in a cardboard box (this was just prior to growing up) with my friend. The box is closed and there is a knock on

101

the side. When we open it, there he is: blonde, blue eyes and gorgeous. And a proper gentleman too, with the good manners to knock.

I am besotted. Wherever he is, I want to be there. He only lives a few doors away from us, yet until now I've not been aware of his existence. Now I become conscious of him all the time.

Soon after this, he begins to call at our house, supposedly because he is a friend of my brother's. But I know better. He's only calling to see me. Of course he is. I keep my secret for as long as I can, which isn't very long. In the end I just have to share my secret and joy with Celia.

I wait for the right moment, which comes one evening when we are both ogling the mirror, as usual. She is getting ready to go out while I am looking for blackheads and pimples, and zapping them, like a young Arnold Schwarzeneger. Oh, to have one of those mirrors which Snow White's stepmother possessed and which gave one not just their reflection, but reassurance as well.

So there we are, my sister and I, arguing as usual, when I say, 'I have a boyfriend, anyway.'

'So have I,' she says

'Who is he then?' I ask

'Who is yours?' she retorts.

I am filled with pride as I tell her his name, having one up on her for once. But my moment of glory is short lived.

'He can't be yours,' she says.

'Why not?' My voice is beginning to tremble.

'Because he's mine,' she says defiantly.

'He can't be,' I say heartbroken.

'Well he is. I've been going out with him for months. Where do you think I'm going now?'

I am devastated. How could he do this to me? All the time I thought he was calling to see me, he was coming to see my sister. Oh, I don't like him very much now, the traitor. Bobby Moore would never have done that to me, though that guy without the teeth – now he's another matter entirely. I vow that the next time I fall in love (in a week or two, I hope) I'll make sure he loves me first.

Despite this resolution, my hormones are still working overtime and I can't help but fancy any likely fella I see. In fact a lot of fancying and being fancied in turn goes on, especially by 'the pole'. This is, in fact, a street light which ironically rarely gives out any light because no sooner has a new bulb been fitted, than those Romeos who don't want their courting with their Juliets spotlighted, smash it.

Now despite the height of this 'pole', many of the young girls around the area are constantly climbing it. Regularly I hear the women in the street whispering to each other, 'Such and such a one is up "the pole".' Whenever I hear this, I run down there as fast as I can to catch this phenomenon. But by the time I get there, they've always climbed back down and disappeared from sight.

I marvel at how the girls can climb 'the pole'. Nearly all of those whom I've heard named, have big bellies on them. Afterwards, most of them are rewarded with a baby for their efforts, but strangely enough, no one ever seems too happy about this.

I think it would have been much easier for those girls to have looked under a head of cabbage for a baby. But it seems they all prefer getting up 'the pole'. It'll only be a matter of time before one falls from the top of it, and then we'll see.

The local fellas congregate by 'the pole' and we girls ensure that we 'just happen' to be passing in our skimpy jumpers and minis when they're there. We think ourselves glamorous, sophisticated and grown up, yet we don't really know why we're parading about like horses in the enclosure before a race. Maybe it's because the fellas call us nice fillies and tell us how much they'd like a ride. You should see the size of some of them. I can tell you, I'm giving none of them a piggy back.

But in our house, our mother doesn't like us girls going to 'the pole', and her advice is always ringing in our ears. 'You mustn't throw yourself at a man,' she says. 'Always respect yourself and you won't end up a fallen woman.'

Since I am so hurt after my falling in love experience, I certainly heed her advice. I am determined I won't throw myself at anyone and certainly not from the top of 'the pole'. No one's going to point at me and say, 'Look at her. She's a fallen woman.' Anyway, knowing my luck, I'd more than likely miss. But I am soon to find, to my cost, that one can be thrown too.

***

I am thrilled when I learn to cycle. It is a hard and difficult task with the bad leg and all, but eventually I get the hang of it. But when I first start out, I find that I am unable to push the pedal with my left leg. It is much too weak for the job. When my sister Kathleen learns of my problem she advises me to try out my big boot. This has long since been discarded, but it is now enlisted to help me learn to cycle.

And it works a treat. Its weight alone is sufficient to push the pedal around and once I get the hang of it, soon I am making progress. I have to adapt to my method by pushing harder with my right leg in order to bring the left pedal up into a vertical position. Then, by momentarily standing on the left pedal, with the weight of the boot, it is forced back down. In this way I am able to cycle. Once I get the hang of it, I become a fully qualified, and competent cyclist. So much so, that I can even discard the boot. Once more, it is banished to the bottom of a press.

Having got quite accomplished at cycling, one evening Theresa allows me to cycle on her bicycle. What is more, she allows me to carry her on the back. I am careering down the street when all the prospective boyfriends are gathered by 'the pole'. Theresa asks me to stop as she wants to talk to them. I think she fancies someone.

As I pull to a stop, she leaps off the bicycle in a great hurry, not even giving me sufficient time to release my right foot from the pedal strap. So I am left stranded with only my left leg supporting me and the bicycle. While Theresa goes off to talk to the boys, it looks like I'm the one who's going to end up a fallen woman.

I scream out her name, aware that my left foot won't support me for more than a second or two, but she ignores my screams, as do the Romeos. I scream yet again, but it is of no use.

Then, almost as though in slow motion, the bicycle and myself topple over. All eyes are now on me as I lie there with the bicycle on top of me. I have their attention now, the swines, when I certainly don't want it.

'What's the matter with you?' they laugh.

'I fell,' I say, but I'm sure no one believes me. They think I am just looking for notice and fall deliberately. Well I was looking for notice but of a different kind.

I free my foot, but I am in no mood now for fancying anyone. After all, I am a young teenager and I've fallen. Teenagers don't fall. Well, maybe they do fall into fellas' arms but certainly not on the ground. My life is ruined. How can I ever face anyone again? I pick myself up, brush my grazed knee and go home. No more fancying for me, I decide, at least for the moment.

As the summer draws to a close, September comes around and school beckons. But it is more of the same – cooking and sewing and washing and ironing – under the guise of Domestic Science. As I don't want to be a Domestic Scientist, I feel it is a waste of time and I leave. But as there are few jobs for failed Domestic Scientists, I find myself wandering the streets. One day, I am with my friend when a suspicious looking man pushing a bicycle stops us. 'Where do ye think ye're going?' he asks with some authority.

I am indignant at his manner and answer cheekily, 'Nowhere'.

'Why aren't ye in school?' he asks.

'Because we've left,' I say, cocky as you like. My friend giggles and I nudge her. I don't like this strange looking man – we really shouldn't even be talking to him, especially as he is wearing a tweed cap, and bicycle clips and looks like a pervert. I don't know what a pervert is apart from the fact that they usually wear dirty raincoats and do a lot of flashing. In fact, I don't really even know what one looks like – but somehow I get the feeling that I might have met one at last. The bicycle is the only complication. I'd never heard that they usually had one but maybe it's the light on the front they flash.

'What's your name?' he now demands angrily.

'Why?'

'Do you know who I am?'

'No,' I say, thinking it might be best not to let on that I think he's a pervert.

'I'm the Schools' Inspector,' he pronounces in a very official sounding voice, 'and ye should both be still at school.' He looks at my friend and then turns to me. 'Whatever about her, you should still be in full time school.'

As my friend giggles uncontrollably, I become indignant again. 'I'm older than her,' I say defiantly, but he doesn't care. He takes our names and a week later our parents are instructed to send us to school on a one-day per week basis, or else. I don't know what the 'else' actually entails, but it works. We are both sent back to school. Here we spend most of our time eating what we are taught to bake, though I am mainly an onlooker in the latter category.

Until the summer holidays in 1967, I attend the one-day-a week school. By now my eating has improved immensely but I still can't bake. My parents haven't been entirely happy with this state of affairs, and so when I leave school officially, and take to wandering the streets again, my mother decides it is time I get a job.

Knowing how shy I am, and aware that I am unlikely to find a job by myself, she obtains one for me as a shop assistant. I am delighted and, though apprehensive, I am determined to work hard and impress my boss.

But I think I impress him a bit too much. Each time we are alone in the shop he crouches down before me and stares at my bosom (which has matured much faster than the rest of me) and becomes breathless, like an asthmatic. I didn't know until then that asthma, which a neighbour thinks I have got, was contagious and that you could get it just by looking at a big chest.

With my having such an adverse effect on this man, I begin to wonder if anyone will ever risk his life by marrying me. My only hope seems to lie with the short sighted, providing, of course, I can keep them far enough away so the eyeful they get is rather hazy and a bit on the small side.

Anyway, I soon realise that I won't be able to keep my boss far enough away if I continue to work in his shop. So I ask my friend for advice. 'He's just a filthy pervert,' she says. 'I think you should leave.' Knowledge at last. So a pervert can simply be a heavy breather too and doesn't even have to own a raincoat or a bicycle. Mind you he'd have problems cycling with lungs like that. Maybe he's just envious of the size of my lungs and would like to have them, unaware that at times I breathe just as heavily as he does.

So after just three days, I leave. On the Friday I go to collect my wages. But as I don't wish to go alone, and my friend has never seen a real pervert, she comes with me. While she stands beside me, giggling as usual, I am paid for my three day's hard labour the princely sum of £1-10s. That's what I am worth – ten bob a day. It's a sobering thought.

But even more sobering is the thought that now I've left my job, I am going to be in the wars again at home. And it will be every bit as bad as the Vietnam war which is reported on the news every day, though out there it seems to be gorillas that are doing most of the shooting and killing. For the life of me, I cannot understand how they trained gorillas to fight. I didn't even realise there were gorillas in that part of the world. I thought they only lived in the African jungle, eating bananas and beating their chests, waiting for the imminent arrival of David Attenborough.

Now with no job to occupy me, and with so much spare time, I decide to turn my hand to writing poetry. But I need a subject, and though I might be ignorant of gorillas, I know a great deal about race horses. For a start, I know they are much safer than gorillas. Horses might bolt or bite or kick or throw you, but I've never heard of a horse shooting anyone. And they earn more than ten bob a day – certainly enough to have their shoes hand-made and their manes combed and tied up with ribbons. Tthe best of them have the added bonus of having Lester Piggott ride them too.

I really dig Lester Piggott and Pat Taffee and Nijinsky and Arkle. But Lester – well, he is something else. I love him. But I am very worried because he never smiles. My brother says it's because he's hungry all the time. Apparently a horse can eat more than a jockey. No wonder other men, who are not jockeys, always get happy when they speak about getting their oats.

Well I feel so sorry for Lester that I decide to begin my great career as a poet by writing a brilliant poem for him. I feel it will help him somehow. It goes like this:

> O, Lester Piggott, why do you look so lonely?
> O, Lester Piggott, why do you look so sad?
> You won every race you entered in.
> But never a smile from you, it's a sin.
>
> Arkle was so proud to have you in his saddle.
> But still not a smile from you, it's a riddle.
> You won every race you entered in,
> But still not a smile from you, it's a sin.

I am very proud of this poem and in no way embarrassed to show it to my brother Tom, who is a great poet himself. Well, I for one, was very impressed with the poem he wrote for his wife when their first daughter was born. It is a wonderful sonnet entitled: 'Shall I compare thee to a summer's day?' I still think it's better than anything Shakespeare wrote, except perhaps for that 'thee' bit. That's just the kind of thing Willie would have stuck in.

So it is that with baited breath I wait for my brother's reaction. He is silent for a while. My great literary work has left him speechless. Not many poets, or poems, can do that. I am beginning to feel ecstatic.

But then he strikes, like a true critic, with ridicule and without mercy. 'That's not very good,' he laughs.

It's my poem, so I have to defend it. 'What's wrong with it?' I demand.

'Well for a start, it's factually inaccurate. Lester Piggott never rode Arkle. Arkle is a jumper. Lester Piggott only races on the flat. Now, if you put in his Derby winner, St Paddy, that would be better.'

'But Saint Paddy doesn't scan properly,' I say. 'It will spoil both the metre and the rhythm of my poem.'

'It's not a poem anyway,' he says. 'It's a load of rubbish.'

In that moment, another great Irish poet is vanquished. But I console myself with the thought that my demise as a poet has left the field open for Seamus Heaney. Does he ever imagine, or even suspect, I wonder, the debt he owes my brother? If only Arkle had been able to run as well as jump ...

15

SHAKING ALL OVER

☙

In 1968, violence seems to erupt all around the world. In the US, Robert Kennedy, the younger brother of former President John F. Kennedy is shot dead. And Martin Luther King, the man who had a dream, is assassinated in Memphis.

There are student riots in Paris led by Red Danny, while in Czechoslovakia the Red Army crush the Prague Spring. The whole world is in chaos and the only answer anyone has is to stick a flower in their hair, keep repeating the phrase, 'peace man', and head for San Francisco.

While all this is going on, I am having to face the fact that I am growing up fast. And there is no sign of love anywhere. But I am determined to seek it out and so attend my first dance. It's called a 'hop' and my vivid imagination gives me a picture of everyone hopping around on one leg (it's my Irish dancing experience coming to the fore). I certainly think I ought to feel at home. Hopalong is about to come of age.

The hall is dingy, but with the flashing lights and the latest pop music blaring at high volume, it seems a magical place where dreams could come true. The girls are here, dressed in their mini skirts, their long, swinging hair shining and glinting. The fellas are here too, across the other side of the hall, dressed in their best suits. Their Beatle boots are highly polished and their long hair is slick with Brylcream. And I think it odd that those who so detested wearing boys' boots should now wear Beatle boots. If only I were a boy my own black boots would be in vogue at last.

The only really incongruous note in this wild gathering is the presence of a priest in his dark suit, hovering about the hall like a black bird of prey. He is here, I discover, to put a stop to any blossoming of free love, rolling your own fags or French kissing.

Dancing though, is permissible, though this dancing seems to entail a strange kind of behaviour. With myself amongst the girls in a group on one side of the hall and the fellas in a group on the other, the music begins, 'If you're going to San Francisco,be sure to wear some flowers in your hair'. Though San Francisco seems a very long way from O'Connell Street in Limerick, I still feel that there is magic here. Then, as if at some hidden signal, the fellas stampede across the floor to ask us girls to dance, and there is a great mellée.

I am so shy and so afraid that I will make a fool of myself, that I refuse many offers, stating that I can't dance, which of course is true. In fact I should be banned from any self-respecting dance hall or hop. But the fact that I can't dance, doesn't stop my friends from encouraging me. 'Nothing to it,' they tell me. 'You just – well kind of shake yourself a bit.'

This at least seems to be true enough. Any idiot could do it – one only has to have the ability to shake – but I am no idiot. What I need is courage. 'No one will take any notice of you,' my friends say. 'Not with this big crowd.'

One fella is very insistent. I feel he will die of a broken heart if I don't dance with him. After all, I think, I might be the girl of his dreams (but he'll wake up soon enough!). His insistence gives me a false sense of hope and pride. I feel like Cinderella, but with two different sized feet wearing the same size slippers. I'm Juliet on her balcony, Elizabeth Taylor as Cleopatra, showing Richard Burton's Mark Anthony, her asp. I'm all of them rolled into one, little old me with this tremendous power over men.

This fella, I think, will do anything for me. If I lose my slipper – well, shoe actually – I just know that he'll pick it up and then search high and hopefully low – until he finds me. If it happens to be the left shoe though, then of course it won't fit properly when he finds me and he'll probably end up marrying my sister who isn't at all ugly.

So now I see him willing to climb balconies for me, willing to buy me diamond rings, willing to defy the biggest asp in the whole world, if only I will dance with him. 'All you've got to do is shake a leg,' he says, smiling. He doesn't say which leg, which at least gives me a sporting chance.

So, shaking all over, even before I get onto the floor, I follow him to join the crowd of gyrating bodies. The hall isn't very brightly lit so no one will notice me, I think – a very foolish thought, as it turns out. This, I feel, is the hardest thing I've ever had to do, but with the music and the lights and the gyrating bodies around me, I soon get into the swing of it, even if unlike everyone else, I can shake but the one leg. When it is over the fella thanks me and I feel elated. I have done it and no one appears to have taken any notice.

Afterwards, still on a high, I retreat to the 'ladies' where the girls usually gather to discuss who they've danced with and whether they should go home with him or not, if they are asked. Most fellas seem to ask a girl if he can walk her home with the immortal statement that he has his bike outside. But the golden rule is that you only allow a fella to walk you home if he has asked you up dancing a minimum of three times. This ensures that it will be quite safe to go with him. Apparently he won't be looking for free love or French kissing, not even a 'shift', whatever that is.

For most of the girls here, the sole object of the dance is to get a fella to walk them home, even if he is pushing his bicycle. Me, I just want to dance. I've had my first one and I'm feeling elated and I want to have more. But my elation isn't to last too long. A girl approaches me and looks me up and down with complete disdain. 'That was your first dance, wasn't it?' she says.

'Yes,' I say.

'I thought so,' she says. 'I could tell by the way you were

shaking.'

Everyone else must have noticed too, including the fellas, for no one asks me to dance again. And I know why. I had gone there looking for my prince but there are no princes to be found at a local hop; there are no princes in Dom's Dance Hall; in fact there are no princes in Ireland. And even if there were any, they would be too busy fighting their way through thick thorn bushes to find their 'sleeping beauty' to be bothered with the likes of me. No knight in shining armour, I realised, was going to climb any tower to rescue me, even if my hair was long enough to be let down and used as a rope.

Some princes, I knew, could be disguised as frogs, awaiting a princess to kiss them. But they would not be easily recognisable, especially for a first timer like me. So they were out. But maybe all those other fellas at this dance, and at other dances as well, were not looking for a princess at all. Maybe they were looking for something else. Only I didn't have the faintest idea what it might be. All I realised for certain was that I didn't have it.

So now I find myself a teenager with spots and insecurities, no boyfriend and a big problem: the fellas don't seem to want to dance with a girl who has a limp. And to think I had thrown away the ball and chain years before. So what am I to do?

I refuse to wear the conventional boot with a lift, which really just consists of a three-inch thick sole and heel. It's ugly and makes me look like a cripple. But I am not a cripple – despite the claims of the Oxford English Dictionary – I am just a bit lopsided, like the leaning tower of Pisa. This is one of the wonders of the world and no one's ever heard anyone suggest putting a big ugly platform beneath it to straighten it out.

So I am determined to be a wonder of the world too. No one is going to straighten me out. I'll remain crooked, but in the meantime I'll have to try and camouflage the fact. So I decide to invent my own lift and I have the brilliant idea of putting the lift inside my shoe. That way no one will see it.

I get a piece of rough timber, and put it into the shoe. It's brilliant. Instantly I become a fast-talking, straight-walking woman. Now I can't wait to model the new me for my friends. 'Notice anything?' I ask.

They, look hard. 'Yeah, you're walking funny,' they say.

'No I'm not. I'm walking straight.'

'So you are. It just looks funny, you walking straight.'

Now I am ready – ready to knock them dead at the next dance. I feel wonderful. It feels lovely to be level for once. I'm brimming with confidence and happiness and maybe this is contagious, but I get offers to dance. If the fellas suspect they might have seen me here before, only a bit lopsided, they probably conclude that the uneven one must have been my identical twin sister.

But it has been a long walk from the bus to the hop and with all this dancing, my foot begins to hurt. The piece of timber is digging into my toes and heel, so that halfway through, when a fella asks me to dance, I am in agony. I don't want to refuse though. This, after all, is what I've wanted and dreamed of.

By now, I can hardly stand, never mind dance. My limp is 100 times worse. As the fella holds me in a slow dance it is a case of the agony and the ecstasy, one of each in either foot. As he tries to keep me upright, he says what no man has ever said before, 'Is there something wrong with your leg?'

'There is,' I think. 'Some idiot has put a lump of timber in my shoe.' So that is the end of that idea. But I'm not completely beaten yet, despite feeling like the coyote in the 'Roadrunner Show'. I'll keep on trying, no matter what.

The following week I try a block of sponge in the boot. It certainly does the trick and I am even once more. It feels lovely and comfortable. I wear it going out on the street and all the men repairing the road by the Hockey Wall, wolf whistle me.

This is a great boost to my morale. But walking about all day, flattens the sponge, so that by evening, I am down by an inch or more. On passing the same workers, one man asks me, 'Have you hurt your leg, love?'

What can I say? No, I've just flattened the sponge. I say nothing.

It reminds me of that darn coyote again. I am back to square one. Nothing for it now, it seems, but acceptance of my lot. I'm not as determined as that old coyote. But then he doesn't have a bad leg. I'm sure he often wishes that the old roadrunner had a bit of a limp. It might give him an even chance of catching him.

***

In July, I reach the ripe old age of seventeen and I want to remain at seventeen forever. I feel it's such a romantic age and even though I have no romance in my life, I am a real romantic at heart. I think I should have been born French. I would feel at home in Paris. After all, I've spent enough time in plaster of paris to be a French citizen. But I don't know the language, and have never even met a French person. In fact, I know nothing about France really, except it's romantic. So I am very intrigued when one of the fellas tells us he has a French letter.

'Can I see it?' I ask.

'No, you can't,' he says.

'Why not?'

'I have it hidden,' he says.

I don't believe for a minute he has one. I mean, who'd be writing to him from France? He'd be lucky enough to get a letter from Ireland.

'Where is it hidden then?' I ask.

'It's in the fold-up of my trousers,' he says.

I look at the fold ups but I can't see how an envelope can fit in there. I can't even see a trace of white. Theresa, who is much bolder than I am, searches the fold ups, and finds this French letter in one of them – only it doesn't look anything like an envelope and I think that the French must have a very funny way of posting letters.

This letter looks like a badly-made balloon. Maybe it's a personal type of airmail, I don't know. Whatever it is, my friend runs off with it and I follow her, the fella shouting at us to come back.

When we get to her house, she blows it up like a balloon. Eventually it bursts and she discards it. For days afterward we go about warily in case we run into the rightful owner of the letter. But when we do meet him he blushes red as a beetroot and passes us without a word.

That autumn, still boyfriend-less, I go blackberry picking with Theresa. I will go anywhere for a big juicy blackberry. Like the prince in *Sleeping Beauty* I push my way through all the brambles to get to the ripest, juiciest berries. Thorns scratch and tear at my skin, and I'm not even going to meet a prince. Or am I?

When we have picked enough, Theresa and I make for home, eating happily as we walk along. We are almost home when I do meet my prince - a boy I like a lot. We stand chatting for a while and all the time his eyes are smiling. He's smiling at me, I think. At last he has noticed me. I float into the house, elated. But when I look in the mirror I find my face is purple from eating the blackberries. It's little wonder I was noticed.

But much worse than blackberry stains is in store for my face, if only I knew it. We are talent spotting one evening in another area, Theresa and my sister and our friends. I am on that bicycle again but this time I am the one being carried. We are speeding down a steep hill, so fast that even a young Sean Kelly wouldn't catch up with us. But hopefully he'd have had brakes on his bicycle.

During this high-speed descent my friend informs me that she has no brakes. Naturally I don't believe her until she pulls both brake levers and nothing happens. Well, that's not strictly true. There is one almighty bang as we crash into the kerb trying to avoid an oncoming bus. I am thrown to the pavement where I lie battered and injured. The flesh on my left arm and leg is torn and bloody and painful, as is my face. But the real pain is caused by the fact that all the fanciful fellas have witnessed the whole incident. My sister runs up, and after taking one look at me, insists I go to the hospital.

'Why?' I ask.

'You haven't seen your face,' she says. 'You can't go home like that.'

After an argument, we set off for the hospital where I am taken into casualty. My sister and friends remain outside. After examining me, the doctor informs me he will have to give me an injection and then clean me up.

'Now, I won't hurt you,' he says.

Naturally he is lying through his teeth. But I agree with him. 'I know you won't,' I say, 'but the needle will.'

I get the injection and it does hurt. Then he sprays something on my arm. The pain is almost unbearable. I moan a little but I do not scream. No one will ever hear me cry. I realise that the pain will be a hundred times worse if I let him near my face with that lethal spray, so I say to him, 'You're not putting that on my face.'

'OK,' he says, smiling reassuringly. 'Just close your eyes, then.'

I do as he asks – I would do anything for him – and the swine sprays my face. But when I open my eyes he is smiling at me and my anger dissolves instantly. 'Now, let's take a look at that knee,' he says. This seems more promising. 'But why is it,' I think, 'that I always have to be in bother before a man wants to look at any part of my body?'

The knee is very swollen but nothing is broken. So it is merely bandaged up and I am released. He is a lovely doctor – maybe he likes me, maybe he has never seen a knee like mine before – but in any event, he comes out to the main door of the hospital with me and, pointing at the less than roadworthy machine, asks, 'Is that the offending bike?'

'Yes,' I say.

'Well, best not get up on it again. It's dangerous without brakes.'

'How do you expect me to get home in my state, then?' I laugh as I perch myself dangerously on the carrier and we set off. He laughs, at my foolishness, as he returns to his work. No doubt he sees many such as me, young, carefree and without a sense of danger. But then we're the ones who keep him in work, so why should he complain?

16

BREATHLESS

☙❧

In order to keep out of trouble, when I am over my ordeal of falling from the bike and being sprayed with toxic substances, I get myself a job – in a hospital. The same hospital where I'd spent some time as a baby and where my parents had to stand on a box to look at me through the window.

The place has hardly changed since then, though of course I don't remember it. For my first duties, I am assigned to the geriatric ward. Remembering my first job, I hope there will be no perverts here who begin panting when they see my bosom. But if there are, at least I should be able to move much faster than them.

My mother has always recommended to us that we do domestic work as our first introduction to the work force. She feels that it's somewhat similar to what in Britain they call 'doing national service', and is a great character builder. 'After you've experienced that,' she tells us, 'everything else will seem easy.' She's certainly right about that, I think, as I begin my career as a domestic. It's very hard work, but surprisingly, I love it.

The hospital duties are Dickensian, as is the hospital itself. David Copperfield had it easy compared to what I've got to endure. It's a 7.30am start, which means leaving home at dawn to walk to the hospital, a most unpleasant experience when it's lashing rain and there's a bitterly cold wind blowing.

The main kitchens are in a separate building to the geriatric wards and it is hard crossing from one to the other on cold or wet mornings, with just a light uniform to protect me from the elements. A large churn of milk, which must last the whole day, and a gigantic pot of porridge – the pot is large enough to boil me whole – have to be wheeled across the yard from these kitchens to the smaller kitchen beside the geriatric ward. The wheels on the trolley are so stiff that it may as well have none. It is the hardest part of the day.

While the porridge is being served up by the sister in the kitchen, I deal with the trays, which have been prepared the previous evening. Three trays are stacked on top of each other with cup, saucer and side plate These have to be carried to the ward and each patient is given one tray. Because I am so small, I have to look through the gap between the trays because I cannot see over the top.

We now serve all the patients with their bowls of porridge and when they've eaten those we give out the buttered bread and tea from huge teapots which look more like kettles. Lastly, there is more tea for those who want it.

With the breakfast over, it is a matter of clearing up and washing the ware. Then there is the soiled linen to be collected and floors to be swept and washed. At eleven, boiled milk is served and no sooner is that dealt with than preparations begin for lunch.

At noon I make another trip across the yard to fetch a large jug of soup, a smaller jug of gravy and a large tray of potatoes. It is a real juggling feat to manage. With the soup in one hand, the gravy in the other and the tray tucked in between my arm and side, I walk across the yard, arms akimbo and leaning to one side like Charles Laughton's Quasimodo in *The Hunchback of Notre Dame*.

I can manage fine on my own, but if there is someone with me, or I meet someone, and either one makes me laugh, then all the shaking causes the potatoes to drop, one by one, to the ground until there are very few left on the tray. Then when I reach the geriatric ward, the sister on duty loudly complains that the kitchen is not sending across sufficient potatoes, and I have to make the trek again. At least it's easier to manage the tray without the two jugs. And now, if I meet someone who makes me laugh, I can just about ensure that I keep enough potatoes on the tray to satisfy the sister and, more importantly, the patients.

We serve up the lunch but now there is the extra course of desert to be given out and I find myself running around trying to get everything done. Then there is the clearing up and washing up to be done and after that, a mountain of bread to be buttered in readiness for the evening tea and the next day's breakfast.

Then, I can have a welcome break for an hour and a half. I usually go home, glad to be out of that grim building for a little while. I have to be back again in time for the tea. In the evening, when I finish for the day, I feel so exhausted that I literally have to drag myself home. My feet ache and when I get home I place them in a basin of water, to soothe them.

Life goes on its uneventful way and I relax. There are no heavy breathers – well, to be strictly honest, there are, but at least they're not breathing heavily because of my big bosom. I am breathing heavily from all the running around, trying to serve them, and perhaps that's why one day, when I have a chore to carry out, I decide to take the easy way out and conserve my lungs. It turns out to be a big mistake.

I have just given the patients their tea when the sister sends me upstairs to one of the other wards to get some extra butter. In a hurry as usual, and thinking to save my lungs on the stairs, I choose the quickest way. I dash into the lift, close the outer door, then close the inner door, and then press the button for the third floor – virtually all at once.

The lift moves about an inch and then jerks to a stop. I am stuck. I press the buttons but the lift will neither go up nor down. I realise now that the outer door isn't fully closed. I need someone outside to close it to set me free.

There is no one about. But being a very calm sort of person

this doesn't bother me at first. When about three days have passed though – well, all right, five minutes or so – I begin to panic and worry. The patients will now be looking for their second cup of tea and I'm not there to give it to them. Will they inform a nurse that I am missing, I wonder? But this seems a forlorn hope. Most of them are senile and won't even realise I am missing.

Time passes – the tea must be getting cold by now – and I think I am running out of air. I knew those big lungs of mine would one day be the death of me. They've used up all the oxygen and now I'm running solely on carbon dioxide.

The lift is tucked around a corner so only someone wise enough to use the stairs or foolish enough to risk a lift that gets stuck, or someone going to the kitchen, will find me. But by then, I will surely be dead.

I bang and bang with all my strength but it is no use. No one can hear me. My short life is almost over, a life burdened by lifts. One day a lift for my shoe and the next day trapped in a lift. I have only got the job and now it seems as though I am going to die, on the job. Even if I survive on the carbon dioxide, I'll die of hunger.

I have just resigned myself to my terrible fate when I catch a glimpse of a nurse halfway up the stairs. I start to bang and bang again and eventually she hears the racket, which, come to think of it, is a miracle of sorts, being as she's a whole twenty feet away from me. 'Who's that?' she calls

'Me!'

'Who's you?' My oxygen levels are zero, my carbon dioxide levels are running down and I'm already wasting away from the hunger, yet she's interested in formalities and wants me to introduce myself!

'Me, Joan,' I manage to gasp, much in the manner of Tarzan, but without the wind to do the 'oohhh aahhh' bit properly.

'What's the matter?' she demands, coming back down the stairs. Do all rescuers interrogate people before they set them free? Do firemen ask, 'is that a fire I see before me?', before they heft you over their shoulders and carry you from the burning building?

'The lift is stuck,' I call out to her.

'How did that happen?'

'I don't know,' I lie.

'I can see now what's wrong,' she says, peering in at me through the gap in the outer door. 'You haven't closed the door properly. Don't you know you must close the door fully before the lift will operate properly?'

'Oh God,' I think, 'why did you send me a know-all?'

'You should be more careful,' she says. 'The lift can be dangerous if you don't operate it properly.'

I don't answer. 'Just let me out,' my mind screams.

She closes the outer door and I jab the button for the ground floor. The lift jerks and stops. Desperate, I thrust the doors open and rush out. Determined never to venture into a lift again, I gasp air into my lungs.

The incident changes my life. I develop liftaphobia. A career in America is now out of the question. It would take me all day to climb up 100 flights of stairs and then I'd have to come back down again. And maybe they don't even have stairs in those skyscrapers which would make getting up to any floor impossible.

***

Towards the end of the year I go from working in a hospital to being an inmate. The breathing difficulties I experienced that day coming from the shop have become, over time, an integral part of my life. I even get used to this state of affairs. No one knows for certain what it is or what causes it and it comes and goes with monotonous regularity. After years of hanging out the window in the middle of the night, gasping for air, and being fine again the next day, it is generally supposed that I have asthma. Now it is about to be officially diagnosed, though the events leading up to this are nearly fatal when I almost die, not of a lack of oxygen, but of embarrassment.

The diagnosis is made under 'blackout' rules. The reason for the blackout is our own fault. Because we get up to so much blackguarding and mischief and noise when we go to bed, every now and then my father removes the bulb from our bedroom. Having found that stamping on the stairs a number of times doesn't bring a lull in the bedlam, as a last resort he removes the bulb. Amazingly, that always works and we soon quieten down and go to sleep, with just a glimmer of light from downstairs.

It is on one such night that it is officially diagnosed that I have asthma. Normally, I get an attack in the middle of the night, but on this occasion it occurs after I've been to see the film, *West Side Story*, one I'm not likely to forget, though for reasons other than how brilliant and sad it was.

I am wheezing as I leave the cinema and finding it difficult to breathe. I do not want to draw attention to myself and so I try to keep up with my friends who are walking rather fast. By the time I reach home, I am gasping. I crawl up the stairs and into bed. But there is no relief – rather the opposite. I have no sooner laid my head on my pillow than I feel I'm suffocating. Frightened, I jump up in the bed, not worried about drawing attention now. It happens so suddenly that I scare the living daylights out of my sisters. 'I'm going to die,' I scream, with what I think is my last breath.

My two sisters jump out of bed and, after consulting my parents, run off to the nearest public telephone to call the doctor. I am hoping that the telephone will not be out of order or they will have to go further and it will be too late when the doctor gets here.

Hours seem to pass before the doctor arrives, though he is actually here before my sisters return. I see him framed in the doorway, his hand reaching for the light switch. But there is no light and it is then I nearly die of embarrassment.

He fumbles his way towards me in the dark, guided only by the wheeze which is now very loud indeed. Still in the dark – in more ways than one – he diagnoses that I have asthma and that there is nothing he can do and is sending me into hospital.

The ambulance arrives and takes me off to the Regional Hospital, where I am immediately admitted.

I can't imagine what they can do here to stop this attack. But then, could I have ever seen myself topless, my chest whistling at a young doctor (he is really only interested in the sound though) and my pulse racing 190 beats to the minute?

Initially I am given oxygen. They can give me anything, I decide, just as long as they help me to get my breath back. Then I am given an injection. It is simply magic. A feeling of fresh air passes across my face and I find I can breathe easily again. It's brilliant. I feel better instantly. But once I do feel better, modesty takes over and I clutch the sheet across my chest just like the film stars do. Well, the doctor may have cured me, but he is getting no more free looks.

I am now sent up to a ward. In the morning I feel even better and am back to my old trick of eyeing up the fellas again, only this time they are doctors and have to hold your hand, gaze into your eyes and examine your chest. As far as I can see, I breathe through my nose or mouth, and it has nothing whatsoever to do with my chest. But they seem convinced that it is the problem, and examine it frequently. So, aside from that little problem, or big one in my case, hospital seems like a great place to meet a man. And they would certainly know what they were getting, though I suppose many of them mightn't want a heavy breather like me.

Hospitals are wonderful places for other reasons too. Why people constantly complain about them and dread them is a mystery to me. I love them, particularly when I'm not ill (the catch is that you usually have to be ill before you find yourself in one).

I love having all my meals served to me, being able to read in bed, and, as a romantic teenager, dashing young doctors to attend to me. It is exactly what the doctor ordered without even knowing it. It's like a holiday, and I will have many such holidays over the coming years.

17

Highs and Lows

☙❧

It is 20 July 1969, the day after my eighteenth birthday. There is great excitement throughout the world, but not because of my birthday. *Apollo 11* has just landed on the moon, and the first man is about to step onto the lunar surface. It is a momentous occasion, history in the making.

It is a big occasion for me too. Mind you I don't make such a fool of myself as Neil Armstrong manages to accomplish, what with him shouting out, 'This is a giant leap for mankind,' when he steps down from the bottom rung of the ladder (about twelve inches at most!) and hops about a bit. It is just as well I'm not officially an adult yet (I have another three years to go) because I venture out to check if I can see the men on the moon. We've always been told that there's one man permanently on the moon, smiling down at us. Just one though, of no known nationality, not three huge Americans in white boiler suits and motorcycle helmets.

Even though it must be a bit crowded up there, I can't see any of them. Maybe they've all been taken short at the same time. Or else they're hiding.

Anyway, with this double historical achievement of the men landing on the moon and I reaching the milestone of eighteen, I am allowed to have a celebratory party – a real drinking party where people are expected to make fools of themselves, and hop about a bit as well.

Because alcohol is so expensive, I am hard pressed to figure out how I can obtain a sufficient amount for a proper party with what little money I possess. But my memory comes to the rescue when I recall that a year earlier my friend and I had made some sloe wine. We'd buried it in the garden and I reckoned it should be well matured by now. Well, whether it is or not, it's well time for it to come up and party.

Finding it, I know, is not going to be easy. And then digging it up without breaking the bottle is going to require a miracle. So first off, I say a prayer to St Anthony, the patron saint of lost things, to help me find it. And then I say another prayer to St Jude, the patron saint of lost causes (there doesn't appear to be a patron saint for not breaking bottles) to ensure I don't break the bottle when I do find it.

Both of these excellent saints, with a little help from me and my spade, come up trumps in the form of a bottle of rather dubious looking liquid. But everything will surely look much better when the mud is washed off. Hopefully all of it is on the outside. But, just in case, I say another prayer to St Jude.

With monetary donations from my friends, I accumulate enough money to buy some food and soft drinks. But in order to appear really affluent, and to impress the fellas, I must have lots of booze (fellas don't come to parties to eat ham sandwiches or drink Nash's lemonade). The sloe wine, I think, will be my saviour, but on sampling it, it tastes and looks vile. It appears that it's beyond even the powers of St. Jude.

I can't afford to waste it though as the amount of actual alcohol I've got looks meagre in the extreme, and so I decide to make a punch out of it. I pour it into a big bowl, lace it with the vodka and gin I've bought and with anything else of an alcoholic nature I can find in the house. This consists of two bottles of stout belonging to my father, which he will search for in vain at the weekend and a small bottle of what my brother tells me is *poitín*, but which my sister swears is some sort of embrocation my mother has for her sore leg. It smells like Sloan's Liniment, but on a democratic decision, based on the fact that we've still an inch to fill in the bowl, in it goes.

On the afternoon of the party I clear out the front room and then paint all the downstairs doors. Alas it is not quick-drying paint, and as all the fellas arrive, looking fab in their latest trendy gear, they seem to be drawn to the still wet and sticky surfaces like flies to flypaper. Soon there seems to be more paint on their clothes than on the doors.

So the ever-dutiful girls (this is in the days before women's liberation reached Limerick) spend their evening trying to clean the boys' jackets with turpentine. If only we'd thought of it, I'm sure the punch would have worked much better.

After destroying their good clothes, I then proceed to give the fellas alcoholic poisoning. After a couple of glasses of the punch, they are hammered. They don't know what is in the bowl, except that there's an awful lot of it. It's potent stuff and even when it's all gone, they still behave like Oliver Twist, and ask for more.

Being a sensible genius, naturally I don't drink (well, some-one has to live to tell the tale) so I am able to keep an eye on things. The party is a great success and it is still remembered fondly as the party of the painted coats. No one remembers the punch, which maybe is just as well.

***

Soon after this I am off on holiday again, thanks to another bad asthmatic attack. But once the attack is over I'm in the best of health again and I feel I can get down to enjoying my holiday. This time though there is to be no holiday for me. Fear, or rather terror, has entered the equation and I realise for the first time that I could die of an attack.

The day after my attack, a young woman is admitted to our ward with asthma. She arrives in the morning and a few hours later she is dead. After her body is taken away, I begin to feel ter-rible. I don't really know what is wrong. My heart is racing and thumping so violently against my rib cage, I feel it is about to smash its way through. It is most uncomfortable and distressing. I can't relax, can't sleep – I can't do anything.

The night nurse becomes very concerned and calls for a doctor. Eventually a young doctor arrives, and he is simply gorgeous. Despite my condition, I can't resist admiring him. He sits on the bed beside me and holds my hand to take my pulse. Oh the joy of it! I no longer feel ill. I feel like a princess in a fairy tale and he is the prince who has come to rescue me. He continues to hold my hand as he speaks to me and tells me in a quiet, gentle voice that I am suffering from shock.

'Your pulse is going pretty fast all right,' he says.

I smile as I think to myself, 'Of course it's going fast – even faster now that you're holding my hand.' Really, doctors should be warned about the behaviour of young girls and the things they get up to in order to attract attention.

Youth, I suppose, is wonderful and by the time the doctor leaves I am feeling much better. I no longer think that I'm going to die. I'm only eighteen, after all. I have my whole life ahead of me. And at least I have a reason now for my racing pulse. I have fallen in love with yet another doctor. Now I decide that I would willingly die for him, failing to see the irony in this. But I am also aware that any other young girl would willingly die for him as well, and that most of them don't have bad legs.

I am fortunate in that there is only one other teenage girl in the ward. But equally unfortunate in that she too is in love with this young doctor, whom I nickname Dr Lovitt. He is tall and handsome and I know that all the nurses fancy him too. But they stand no chance. Doctors only like sick women.

My rival has an illness which causes her to fall down. One morning, as Dr Lovitt is just about to enter the ward, she happens to be walking out to the bathroom. I watch her and I know what's going to happen next, as if I have already seen this scene in a film. Maybe she has seen the same film because just as she reaches the doctor, she swoons. It's straight out of Jane Austen, but definitely not *Sense and Sensibility*.

The doctor is quick and catches her before she falls to the floor. I am green with envy and wishing it was me. But knowing my luck, he'd probably have let me fall. I am greener still as he picks her up in his arms and carries her tenderly to her bed. It all looks so wonderful.

But when he lays her down on her bed, instead of following the script and kissing her, he slaps her hand hard and tells her not to be a silly girl. I'm relieved now that I hadn't pulled that stunt, though the first bit would have been worth it. All I'm ever going to get is my hand held while my pulse is being taken. Ah well, I can always dream.

***

Through all this time, asthma is not my only problem. Now I find myself worried that I don't seem to be growing upwards at the same rate as I'm growing outwards, and I have only three years remaining in which to gain another few valuable inches. Celia is in a similar predicament – it seems to run in the family.

Anyway we decide to do something about it and write to a height specialist in London. We get, by return, a reply saying that if we send off a certain sum of money, the secret of how to be taller will be ours. So we send off the money and we get – a book! It isn't even a thick book that we could stand up on and at least gain a few inches that way. It is just a little thin book for desperate little people with little brains, written by a man with big ideas about how to make big money the easy way.

The instructions consist mainly of stretching exercises which involve placing our hands as high up on the wall as we can reach – which, come to think of it, isn't all that very high. There are no instructions on when we should stop reaching upwards with our hands, but we suppose that when we eventually touch the ceiling, we'll have to stop anyway. By then, we should be tall enough for anything.

These exercises drive us up the wall in more ways than one. And though we gain no extra inches in height, we do end up with what must be the longest arms in Ireland. Often during this fruitless exercise I find myself wondering how tall the height specialist is and guess that he is more than likely a midget, and the only thing he ever increased was his bank balance.

After a few weeks, we give up the exercises. A kind friend, who must have a penchant for sadism, suggests the rack as being the most likely remedy now. But as racks aren't freely available - not even on mail order from unscrupulous midgets – we have to give that one a miss.

After these abortive attempts, it is back to camouflage again. My sister is able to wear high heels so she can gain some extra inches that way. It's difficult for me to wear high heels, but not entirely impossible. Whenever I wear them though, it is a case again of the agony and the ecstasy which I've already endured in a desperate attempt to get even.

Many girls I know go some way to solving this problem by having their hair styled in a bun. The smaller they are, the taller they have the bun. Sometimes, with the high heels and the hair put together, there is only 50 per cent of the person in between.

But I suffer for my extra inches and will continue to do so until I get sense. Walking in high heels is bad enough, but then falling off is quite another matter. And as this looks much worse than the limp itself, or being small, I decide it is time for a change. According to Charles Darwin, we evolve over time. So I decide I will try to evolve, only over a short period. I can't be waiting about for millions of years.

So I begin to walk with the long leg in the road and the short leg on the pavement. This makes me appear even. But I find out that it is a dangerous matter and I have to be vigilant or I will be run over by the cars and lorries and buses whose drivers hurl abuse at me and scream at me to get off the road – which, I think, is unfair as I am only using about four inches of road anyway. No wonder evolution has taken so long, with all the ignorant people about.

But I am only a blink of time into my evolutionary stage when I encounter a problem. 'Is there something wrong with your leg?' a new recruit to our group of friends asks me, as we stroll along.

'Yes,' I reply. Evolution doesn't seem to be working so I decide to get back onto the pavement with both feet.

'Gosh,' she says, when I do so and we're strolling along again. 'You wouldn't even notice it.'

So I have evolved! This girl only noticed me limping when I wasn't limping. Now that I am limping, she claims she hardly notices me. Another few weeks evolving and I'll be perfect. But alas, it isn't going to be, for I find the pavement is a little too high for comfort and walking half on it and half on the road is putting a strain on my muscles and joints. I think about asking the city council to lower the pavement to exactly two and a half inches. But even for them to come to a decision would take millions of years alone. So I am back to square one.

All this is getting me down, while my leg continues to let me down – more often than not right in the centre of the city when there is an audience to enjoy the spectacle. It is most embarrassing. So faced with this problem, there are two things I can do. I can fall under it all, which I do frequently, or pretend it is a war injury and get tough.

I get tough.

As luck would have it, the next time I am admitted to hospital with yet another asthmatic attack, I hear the doctors whispering among themselves about putting me on steroids. They must be considering sending me to the Olympic Games, I think, and I begin to imagine the sort of muscles I will get.

So you can imagine my disappointment, some days later, when the doctors change their minds and decide not to put me on the steroids after all. Not only will there be no gold medals for Ireland, but I will remain a puny lady. But real ladies don't limp. Real gentlemen, on the other hand, and tough men too, can limp and can even look attractive while doing it.

So I pretend that I am tough and decide that my mentor

should be Clint Eastwood. With a glint in my eye, my hips swaggering and my thumbs hooked in the waist band of my jeans, I am ready to draw. I practice for hours with my brother's toy gun, drawing fast and then twirling it about on my finger. I am a real tough guy at last, ready for anyone and anything. But unknown to me, my tough guy image is about to be tested.

It happens at a mixed dance where older men and women (they are at least 40 years old) gather along with teenagers. We go along only for the craic. We do not want to dance with any of these geriatrics who've never heard 'The Hippy Hippy Shakes'. Indeed, anyone over 25 is ancient in our eyes.

Though I don't have the cigar, I am not armed and there is no stubble on my face, I'm still pretty tough and not ready to be messed with. So when one of the old men (at least 50 if he's a day) asks me to dance I refuse, and quite rightly too I think. After all, he's almost certainly married and I've heard that married men are only after one thing. But he isn't getting his hands on my Magnum.

When I refuse, he shakes his fist at me, in jest I suppose, but I take this threat very seriously. And Theresa's reaction doesn't help matters. 'Are you going to let him get away with that?' she demands.

'What can I do?' I ask.

'Go up to him and tell him off.'

'I can't.'

'I thought you were tough,' she says, 'and would do anything for a dare.'

'I am,' I say, 'and I would.'

'Well, I dare you,' she eggs me on.

There is no way out. But I know that I can't do it as wee Joan. So Clint Eastwood it has to be. It takes a few minutes to change from an attractive woman, seeking handsome men to woo her, into Clint Eastwood, who only has to stand there to attract women and frighten men.

Now I am ready to strike terror into the heart of this man who has done much worse than simply laugh at my mule. But after I've dealt with him, he won't threaten me again. There he stands against the wall, with his three friends.

He is totally unaware of the danger as I approach, a cold glint in my eye, my thumbs hooked menacingly in my pockets. I stride up to that bunch of no-good dudes, real cool, with no fear whatsoever in my bones, and burst in on their conversation. I look up at the hombre, (it's a long way up) and say menacingly, 'Watch who you're threatening'.

They stop talking and look at me, dazed and stunned. I've done it – I've frightened them. There will be no more harassment now – no more shaking of fists. No one speaks – they are too scared to. Silence seems to echo through the hall. I think I hear the bar being cleared as people scramble to get out of the line of fire. Others are leaving. I can even sense their fear.

Then suddenly and without warning the four burst out ... laughing. They actually laugh at me, Clint Eastwood. I stare at them, thinking how lucky they are that they hadn't laughed at my mule. All my friends laugh too. They think it's a great joke. But it's no joke to me. For me, it's real. I have done it. I have conquered my fears and boldly threatened four grown men. But in my moment of triumph, I am about to be struck down.

The cold night air after the heat and smoke in the dance hall takes its toll on me. I become very ill with the asthma shortly after getting home and once more I am rushed to hospital. Here, after the usual magical injection, I again feel fine.

After the usual few days I'm told I can go home. But later, a nurse informs me that I cannot go home yet. It appears I have to have a screen test. I ask her what a screen test is, but she will not tell me. Some other patient says that you're placed in some sort of box and whirled about so as to test everything. I wake the following morning with another attack, the first time this has happened while I'm in the hospital.

Despite this ominous occurrence, I rally fairly quickly when a young but very tired doctor administers to me. Then I am told that I can go home in two days time. No one comes in to take me home though so I have to stay another night.

Now it really becomes scary. The following morning I have yet another attack. But again I recover. The next day is Saturday and I am determined to go home, otherwise I will never get out of here. And I desperately want to go to the Saturday night hop.

My brother Pat and a friend of his arrive to see me. They are riding bicycles but that will do me. I am discharged and off I go, waving happily to the nurses as we whiz away. I have been cooped up for a whole week and I am determined to go out against all parental advice. But then we teenagers know it all. I know I won't get sick again. I'm fine. I'm perfectly well enough to go to the hop. And to the hop I go.

Sunday morning it's gasp, gasp, gasp yet again. I cannot believe it. I do not want to go to hospital any more. I'm fed up of all the holidays. And anyway, fellas are much more important than holidays. And so I fight the attack all day long.

Each breath gets harder and harder until I think I can stand it no more. Eventually I collapse. People rush into the house and I am drenched in holy water, reminding me of that day in Knock which seems so long ago now. The ambulance is called but there is no way I can walk even the few yards to where it stands outside the house.

For a moment, I open my eyes and glance up into the handsome face of a young prince. And then I close my eyes again as he sweeps me up into his arms and carries me to the ambulance. It only takes a few seconds but it feels great. Who needs air, not that I'm getting any? And what little I've got, he's taken away. I now fully appreciate the saying, 'take your breath away'.

The siren goes on and I am on my way to the hospital, this time accompanied by my mother and father. But I am much too ill to understand the significance of this. At the hospital I am given the magic injection, but this time it doesn't work and I am put in the corner by the door, the screens pulled about me. This is where the people who are dying are put.

Is this it I think? I am only eighteen years of age. I have not really lived yet. Through the night I am given oxygen and I pity the smokers who cannot smoke. I lie flat against the pillow, wondering whether I am still alive. I stare at a crucifix hanging above the door and I reason that I must still be alive if I can see that. I lie perfectly still, afraid to move, as it is better not to exert myself. Eventually, I sleep.

I wake at about six the following morning and I am aware that it is easier to breathe. I am lying in exactly the same position as I was before I fell asleep. Now I remain like that, afraid even to move my head or sit up, in case the attack returns. I know I've had a fright and I vow that never again will I allow an attack to progress so far.

A week later I am fine and out in the world again. I'm back to my old self, but suddenly reminded of how close I came to dying when a man salutes me in surprise and shock as I get off the bus. 'I thought you were dead,' he says.

'Well I'm not,' I laugh.

'But weren't you bad?' he asks. 'At death's door, I heard.'

'Oh yes,' I say. 'But I'm fine again now.'

And I will be fine from now on, I promise myself, now that I am aware of the danger of an asthmatic attack and now that I know what I have to do. There's no point being a hero where asthma is concerned. The earlier the attack is treated the easier it is for everyone to deal with, including the doctors. But without my being unaware of it, help is at hand. Someone, somewhere is inventing something that will change my life. I'm about to say hello to an Intal inhaler.

18

Love Letters

❦

It is 1970 and a new hop starts on a Saturday night that we are allowed to attend. This suits Hopalong Cassidy fine (well, it is a bit tame for Clint Eastwood) except no one wants to dance with me. So while I don't actually enjoy the hop, I love the music and live in hope that one day my prince will be there, waiting for me, complete with pumpkin, footmen and a spare slipper.

Each Saturday, just like Cinderella, I have to clean the house. I have two sisters, who do not happen to be ugly, and who don't do any cleaning either. Should a prince bearing a glass slipper come looking for me on a Saturday, he will find me washing the wooden stairs with a scrubbing brush, a basin of soapy water and a piece of rag for mopping up. When he's seen my two black knees, if he's still inclined to try the slipper on me, it more than likely won't fit.

This is how I look one Saturday evening when I answer the door to come face to face with the one I loved – he who loved another – the swine. He greets me with amused laughter and it's lucky for him he doesn't have a glass slipper with him or I would have broken it over his head. He might laugh now, but if he sees me in a few hours time, he won't recognise me.

After the tea I go off to clean myself up, a ritual I mostly love. First of all, I wash my hair at the kitchen sink and then try to cajole someone to rinse it for me with luke-warm water from a jug. That done, I now need a bath, especially to clean those black knees. But it is very difficult to have a bath when we haven't got a bath and so I have to make do with a plastic basin filled with hot water, a sponge and a bar of Palmolive soap. These are taken to the privacy of the bedroom where, as I sponge myself down, I dream of one day having a real bath.

After the blanket bath, I iron my hair, a very difficult process. I have this wild curly hair, which most women seem to spend a fortune trying to attain. Me? Well, I just want to have long dark straight hair. So with my head tilted sideways and the hair spread out on the ironing board, I do my best with the electric iron on its lowest setting to straighten out the curls. Even on this setting, the iron gets quite hot and I have to be careful not to singe the hair or burn my face.

With the ironing complete, I now put on my make up: hide and heal for all the pimples. Foundation – Sheer Genius, of course – then mascara and lipstick. I slip into my multi-coloured mini dress and hey presto! Cinderella is ready to go to the hop, where alas she doesn't have a ball.

The prince never shows up, which is just as well. I don't think he'd comprehend a priest walking around separating the young couples who are dancing too close, by tapping them on the shoulder with a cane. Any prince who got hold of a girl's leg to try on a glass slipper would definitely get thrown out.

Despite my disappointment at the failure of my prince charming to turn up, I still look forward to the Saturday night hops. But these, like so many other activities, turn out to be detrimental to my health. One Saturday night, I arrive home breathless and now instead of sending for the doctor, my sisters call the ambulance and again I find myself in hospital.

I do not have the usual Irish doctor to attend me. Instead I have a very large, foreign doctor. And while I lie gasping, he entwines both his hands as though he is about to crack his knuckles, and presses down hard on my chest. What little air I have in my lungs is expelled, and now I don't even have enough breath to call him a pervert.

But he is kind and understanding and I forgive him, especially when he tells me he might be able to do something to help me. So this turns out to be one visit to the hospital I won't regret. For when the attack has been brought under control and I'm about to be discharged, the doctors inform me they are going to give me an inhaler to try out at home. A capsule filled with powder is placed in this inhaler, which looks like the mouth piece for a musical instrument. I must click some section of this contraption, place it in my mouth, and unlike a musical instrument, I must suck instead of blow – which is all very well when you have your breath, but what happens when you can neither suck nor blow?

This, I am told though, is a preventative. I must take it regularly, even when I'm fine, and it will prevent me having an attack. This sounds too good to be true, but I am willing to try anything if it'll keep me well.

Like the magic injection, it works. Even when I'm in a smoky atmosphere, I don't get an attack. After a while I become blasé and think I'm cured and stop using it. And then one night I feel my chest tightening up. The doctors have warned me that by this point it's too late to take the inhaler, but when did I ever listen to advice?

I take the inhaler with what little breath I have, wondering what excuse I can give the doctors for ending up with an attack. I wait with trepidation and within minutes I feel relief. I can't believe it. The inhaler has worked. Within half an hour I'm fine. Now that I can control my attacks, a great weight has been lifted from my shoulders.

Now I decide I must find out all I can about this illness. So I go along to the library and read up on it. The first thing I come across is that asthma occurs mostly at night. But I don't need to be told that. How many nights have I spent gasping in my bed? And in the end, tired and exhausted, have to resort to placing a pillow on the window sill, laying my head uneasily on it, and sucking in all the air I feel is out there in the great big world. I also learn that breathing difficulties get much worse in the middle of the night and towards the dawn, but no one really knows why.

I think I know the reason for this, but do not publish my findings in *The Lancet*. They wouldn't believe me anyway. I already know that we breathe in oxygen and breathe out carbon dioxide. Trees on the other hand, do it the other way round. But at night the trees take in oxygen, so it stands to reason that at night, there is less oxygen about.

So all those times when I've been gasping and hanging out the window for fresh air, there was probably much more fresh air in the room. The discovery doesn't really help my asthma though. And anyway, the air outside the window still feels better – it is cool and soothing, and I feel as if it's getting down deep into my lungs. While I have that feeling, the fear is banished.

Those who have never experienced difficulty in breathing cannot understand the terror of not being able to breathe. During those times when it seems as if I will never be able to take another breath, when my mouth is wide open and there is still no air to be had, then it is truly terrifying. There is nothing I can do and so I cry, and it seems like the crying helps me to breathe.

Because of the frequency of the attacks I've had, and because we live in an old damp house, the doctors advise us to move. New corporation houses are being built on the southside of the city and one of them would be much more suitable for us. There is a great deal of discussion about the merits of this. My father isn't so sure about such a move and he points out the many negative points of doing so. My mother, on the other hand, is all in favour. She still hates this house and Killeely, and can't wait to get away.

I don't want to move either. This is my home and my friends live nearby. If we move to this new housing estate, we'll end up miles from here. But my mother's determination prevails and me and my asthma are great levers for her to use to get her own way. Within months we move to a brand new terraced house on the other side of the city.

The most positive aspect of this new house for me is that it has a bathroom with a real bath. For years I have longed for a bath and at last I've got one. It's simply wonderful. I can't wait for the water to be heated from the boiler at the back of the open fire and then climb into a bath of steaming water, to lie down and close my eyes and imagine I'm in heaven. It is heaven too and I don't ever want to get out, even when the water goes cold. I could just lie there forever.

As well as the wonderful bathroom, the house has four bedrooms, a kitchen and a sitting room. On the outside there's an open porch which is shared with the adjoining house. We all have ideas on how we should go about making the house into a home, but one of my ideas is the only one which meets with serious opposition.

I'm determined to make this new house into a nice home and decide that a pretty lantern fitted to our part of the porch would look terribly grand. No one objects to this, and so a lantern is bought and fitted.

Then, remembering the words of the song, 'Hickory Holler's Tramp', 'The path was beaten wide from footsteps leading to our cabin, Above the door there burned a scarlet lamp', I have the brilliant idea of putting a red bulb in the lantern. If it worked in attracting men in 'Hickory Holler', then it could work equally well here.

But all hell breaks loose at this suggestion. I try to point out that I think it will look nice and homely, omitting my hope that it won't dazzle the many suitors I'm confident will beat a path here to see me now we've moved up in the world. I decide to keep this bit to myself.

The amount of opposition to this idea from my parents though is simply overwhelming. I ask them why they object to the red bulb, but they will only say that you can't have a red light on the house. 'It will attract men to the place,' my mother points out.

'But that's the whole idea,' I want to say, yet wisely I keep silent.

There is much muttering about how the house will look like a place of ill repute and that men will think that it is filled with ladies of the night. And anyway, what will the neighbours think? But in the end I get my way and a red bulb is fitted. How could I have imagined how successful my little ploy is to be? Soon there are enough fellas hanging around our gate to satisfy all the girls in the area, never mind my own meagre requirements. But alas, none of them seem to have eyes for me.

One night, shortly after the bulb is fitted, I am awakened from 'a midsummer night's dream' by a noise outside my window. Within seconds I'm sitting up in the bed, wide awake and alert. Fearless, I get out of bed, pull open the curtain a little and peer out. On the other side of the glass there is a male face peering in at me. Shakespeare might have Juliet calling out, 'Romeo, Romeo, wherefore art thou Romeo?' But I keep my mouth shut. This is no Romeo standing out on the balcony, gazing lovingly in at me. This is a pervert crouched on top of the porch!

Well, he can stay there, I think to myself. So I close the curtains and get back into bed. Thwarted in his attempt to woo one Juliet, he now goes over to the other side of the porch and, looking in the window next door, starts calling out to what he hopes is a more willing paramour, 'Come here. Come here. Hey, come here.'

He doesn't know, of course, that the next door house is built the opposite way about. Here, it is the parent's bedroom he is looking into and it is an angry and irate male face that glares out at him when the curtains are drawn back. I hear his screech of fear, a thump and a cry of pain as he leaps from the porch into the garden, right into the centre of a rose bush.

The next morning the neighbour comes and tells my father what happened the previous night. 'That's it,' my father says in that voice which bodes no opposition. 'That red bulb's coming out.' And out it comes, never to be replaced.

***

Although it is a newly-built housing estate, the people who have been moved here, like ourselves, have come from the poorer, older parts of the city and of course aren't too well off. So around here, a car is still a rarity.

We still have our dreams – dreams which embrace open sportscars – Triumph Spitfires, MG Midgets (which might have been made especially for me) and luxurious limousines. They certainly do not include Morris Minors.

I have a love-hate relationship with this particular car. It looks so sensible, so like a car should, and in black couldn't be anything else but a priest's car. So it seems natural that our young curate should own a black one.

One evening my sister and I meet him while he is putting up posters on the electric poles advertising bingo sessions. We stop to chat to him and he asks us what we're doing.

'Nothing, Father,' I say.

'We're bored, Father,' Celia adds.

'Young girls like ye shouldn't be bored,' he says.

'We have nothing to do, Father,' Celia says. She looks at the Morris Minor. 'Now if we had a car ...' she says mischievously.

'You see that car,' the priest says. 'If I didn't need that car, I'd burn it.'

'So would I,' Celia says. 'Even if I did need it.'

He takes this in good humour and asks us, 'Would ye like to go for a spin? I could do with a hand putting up these posters.' Would we like to go for a spin! Morris Minor or not, we are game.

But it is to be a great disappointment. From pole to pole we speed, in first gear, reaching speeds on one or two occasions in excess of five miles an hour. After a dozen or so poles we decide we've had enough, make our excuses and scarper. We laugh so much at our adventure that we forget how bored we've been.

***

I had thought that the new house would bring changes in my life – especially in my love life – but the arrival of 1971 sees me still without a boyfriend. I am getting old and desperate. My sister, who has a pen friend in India, suggests I find a pen friend for myself. It seems everyone has one these days. So why not me? Through writing, he could get to know me intellectually first. Once he'd got to appreciate my brain, hopefully he'd come to appreciate the rest of me (though I've always believed that any man who goes for brains before curves in a woman needs his head examined).

This solution to my problem works much quicker than I could even dare to hope. A few days later, my sister gives me a torn piece of newspaper with details of a young man in London who is seeking a pen friend in Ireland. Summoning up all my courage, I write to him with vital information about myself. I tell him that I am between four feet eight and four feet ten inches in height, depending on which leg I am standing on when the measurement is taken. I have two long arms (both equal) from desperate attempts to be between five feet two and five feet four inches in height. I also tell him that I once had polio but now only have a bad chest (I include no details of size here except to point out that if my height was in direct proportion to the size of my chest, I'd be at least eight feet tall standing on either leg).

I also inform him that I have long brown hair (length dependant on whether I've ironed it or not) green eyes, and do not believe in Sex Before Marriage. On mature reflection, I'd decided to leave out the intellectual bits until a later letter. I didn't want to put him off, though after posting the letter, I think if he writes back he'll be well worth hanging onto.

Three weeks later he does write back. He says that he found my letter very interesting (it didn't need much deduction on my part to work out which bits they were) he was sorry that I had a bad chest and could I elaborate a bit more on the Sex Before Marriage and why I'd used capital letters. He never mentions my brown hair (ironed or not) nor green eyes, nor the polio, so I know his hormones are all in the right place. I am in ecstasy. Here is a fella who knows what he wants and more important, what he can have.

He begins to take over my whole time – my life. He sends me

143

his photograph – there are two other fellas and a girl in it – all in glorious Technicolor. It instantly becomes the most ravished photo of any fella in history, though it isn't until I later read the enclosed letter that I discover I've been ravishing the wrong fella.

I decide to return the compliment, but being aware of my own reaction to his picture I begin to wonder what he might do with it, or to it. So to be on the safe side I send him a black and white passport-type photograph of myself alone. It is just a head and shoulders picture in case he should have dishonourable intentions. Well, you can't be up to men, now can you?

The photo passes the litmus test. A month passes. Letters are becoming more and more frequent until we are writing daily. By now the intellectual aspects have been well and truly dealt with and he tells me that my brain seems perfectly suitable for him and could he now see what goes with it, the bad bits and the big bits, in fact the whole lot.

This is getting quite serious. I realise now that I will have to send him a full length coloured photograph – in a mini skirt – with both legs on display. This is the part where most of the fellas I've known have found me unattractive. Once they realise that I have an assortment of legs, they vanish. So I know that this will be make or break time. He might not mind the bad chest – that at least will be covered up – but how would he react to the bad leg? Well, at least he can play spot the difference.

I don't really know how to go about getting a proper photograph. I only know how to get passport photos taken in the booth at the railway station. And I don't even have a passport. I have never been outside Ireland. Indeed I would not have been outside Limerick had it not been for the polio. It, at the very least, has enabled me to travel to Dublin, to Croom and to Knock. But despite being so well travelled, I am still very innocent, very green. I haven't ever heard of photographic studios.

But that Christmas Santa Claus is in the city, and so am I. I know I can get a photograph taken there. So off I go to see Santa. I think that no one I know will see me there. I haven't reckoned on meeting my young niece who watches me with amazement from the doorway of Santa's den. Neither had I reckoned on making Santa's day when I stand beside him and he puts his arm about my waist. It is the most pleasurable 'Ho Ho Ho' I've ever heard.

I send off the photograph and I wait expectantly, and not with a little fear, for a reply. Every day I watch for the postman, but of course the first letters I now receive have been written and posted before the photograph could have even arrived in London. And then one day, no letter arrives and I now know for certain that he must have received the photograph and is having second thoughts. When no letter comes the next day I am convinced that this is so.

It is the weekend and there will be no mail until Monday. I am miserable and when Monday comes and there is still no letter, I am devastated. It is going to be a rotten Christmas. So what's new?

On Tuesday, I deliberately avoid the postman and go into town. Here I wander aimlessly through the shops, trying to be oblivious to the Christmas atmosphere. At one stage I am tempted to go back in to see Santa and kick him on the shins just to hear him go, 'Oh Oh Oh' for a change.

When the shops close I have no choice but to go home. There is no spring in my step and no spark in my soul as I enter the house. Someone tells me that there are some Christmas cards for me. There is no mention of a letter or a card with an English stamp.

I pick up the cards, all in large envelopes, and as I flick through them, find a smaller one among them. There is no mistaking the writing or the English stamp. I run straight to my bedroom before opening it – I don't want to break down now in front of the family.

It is the most terrible moment of my life as I tear open the envelope. It is a long letter – I can see that from the number of sheets of notepaper – and I begin to have some small hope. If he didn't want to write any more he'd hardly take six pages to tell me.

It begins, 'My Darling Joan'. This sounds promising. The remainder is in the same vein. The poor fella sounds shell shocked. He says my photograph is the best Christmas present he's ever received, and he can see why Santa has such a big smile on his face. He never mentions the bad leg or the good one for that matter, and so I think that maybe he didn't actually get down past the bad chest. Whether he has or not, it is obvious that he is in love – with me. And so am I – in love with him.

When I recover I notice from the dates that my letter with the photograph and his reply have both been held up in the Christmas rush. All that misery was for nothing. I think about suing the post office but you can't sue anyone when you're sitting on Cloud Nine.

What he also mentions in the letter is that he is sending me a present. He doesn't say what it is – it is to be a surprise. So now I have to endure all that waiting over again. Yet again, the post office lets me down so I have plenty of time to imagine what the present might be. I think it might be a hair brush set – he said he'd love to brush my hair, among other things (obviously not a man for the ironing though) or maybe some jewellery. Or perhaps a watch. I don't have a watch but I don't think I've mentioned that to him.

A few days later it arrives. The parcel is too big and too heavy to be jewellery or a watch. It has to be the hair dressing set. There is no rushing off to the bedroom on this occasion – I am surrounded by an expectant family who seem even more anxious than I am to see what is in the parcel. Presents do not arrive in the post in our house.

I tear open the wrapping paper to find a box underneath which proclaims: Philip's Cassette Recorder. There is a picture on the box of some gadget in a black leatherette case. No one knows what it is. This is turning out not to be a surprise, but a mystery.

I open the box and remove the gadget, still in its case. Someone suggests it is a radio but it has no dials or aerial. Someone else says it is only part of a tape recorder and we begin to wonder when the remainder of it will arrive. So I put it down on the table and we all stand and gaze at it. It must be the most gazed at present anyone has ever received.

The mystery is eventually solved, if not actually resolved, when my brother Mikey arrives home from school. He says it is one of the latest types of tape recorder. I have never seen a tape recorder like this. The only ones I have seen were great big open reel recorders.

Mikey says he knows how to operate it. But the machine refuses to play the small tape, which he says is called a cassette and which has come with it. There is a label on either side of this cassette. On the label on one side is written, 'For you only, Joan', and on the other side, 'Music'. But the machine refuses to do anything for my brother except sit there in silence.

He now proclaims that it is faulty and I should take it into town to have it repaired. This I do the following day. The repair man checks it out and says that it only requires new batteries. He fits these and then shows me how to operate it. I can't wait to get home and play the tape and hear what, 'For you only, Joan', contains.

It is him! I feel weak at the sound of his voice. It is as if he is here beside me. But all my romantic thoughts are quickly banished by my laughter, for the first thing on the tape is instructions on how to play it. One thing is certain. He is definitely an Irishman. Boy, do I love him just then.

The remainder of the tape is first class – all sorts of endearments and protestations of love and wonder at my existence. I begin to realise that love really is blind for not only has he not noticed my leg, but he appears not to have even noticed my chest. But he will – eventually.

The less said about the music though, the better.

19

PLATO'S CHAIR

❦

Well, after receiving such an expensive Christmas present, I decide that this penfriend, whom I've nicknamed Mac, possesses all the ingredients and credentials for a suitable boyfriend for me and so I make sure that I continue writing to him as 1972 begins. Although he lives in London, he comes from Mayo in the west of Ireland, not too far from Knock, as it happens. And he must have once known Mae West, for he promises to come and 'see me some time' during the year.

This precipitates a major crisis when I realise that I don't have any decent clothes in which I might be wooed. I've already made up my mind that I will need a lot of wooing. There will be no 'hands on experience' on our first dates. After all, I have my reputation to uphold and I am at heart a good Catholic girl.

With wooing clothes a priority, I need to find work and fast. But the process turns out to be slow and frustrating. Everything seems to go against me. For a start, I have very little work experience – three days being stared at in a shop, six months as a domestic in the hospital with ten minutes or so stuck in the lift and a stint in the office of a clothing factory – are hardly the best credentials to offer a prospective employer. Add to that the fact that I've had polio and now have asthma, it soon is obvious to me that no one wants a lopsided, heavy breather.

I realise that there is only one solution to this problem – I'll have to be economical with the truth and with the oxygen. So when I am called for an interview at a local rubber factory, I walk fast and talk fast and breathe real slow. I think the interviewer is puzzled by this and asks outright if there is anything wrong with me. 'Oh, I used to have polio,' I say lightly, finding myself unable to lie outright, 'but I'm all right now.'

'That's not a problem,' he says. 'Now if you happened to have asthma or that, what with all the talc in here, that would be a major problem.'

'Really,' I say, taking slow deep breaths, expanding my chest so he can see for himself how big my lungs are. Talc isn't going to be any problem for me, I imply, but from the look on his face I realise that my antics are a major problem for him. Now he's the one doing the heavy breathing, just like my first employer. But he still manages to gasp out, 'You've got the job.'

The next day I find myself employed in the laboratory as the assistant to the laboratory technician, Peg. Here I am to test the rubber which will used in the manufacture of underwear and golf balls. It is a very odd pairing. In the matter of the underwear, the rubber is supposed to prevent the garments from going anywhere – like falling down for instance; while in the matter of the golf balls, it's meant to help them go as far as possible. Obviously it is very important not to get the two types of rubber mixed up. Otherwise we could have Lee Trevino's underpants falling down at a crucial moment while his ball goes nowhere at all.

The work is very interesting – in an odd sort of way. Now I can never watch a golfer on television without wondering if he is using my rubber, in one way or another. I settle in quickly and easily and am only employed about a week when I am faced with my first dilemma. Indeed, it is more than a dilemma for I am actually worried sick when Peg sends me to the guillotine. She tells me that it is situated outside 'despatch', and that they are expecting me and to take a cardboard box with me – presumably for my head.

I have just returned from lunch, and was only a minute late

so feel it is a bit severe to be sent to the guillotine. I haven't even been aware until now that Ireland possesses one. But if factories are installing them, then a great improvement in timekeeping is assured.

On seeing my look of horror, Peg assures me that it is just a small guillotine. But it fails to console me because I only have a small head. I walk slowly through the factory to despatch, but when I get there, I cannot see a guillotine. Naturally I have been looking upwards – I know it is a great big gadget with a blade at the top – having once seen a *Tale of Two Cities* in which Sydney Carton loses his head.

At the time I must admit that I thought that the French revolutionaries might have let him go. Yet what else could they do to shut him up but to chop off his head when he started spouting all that nonsense about it being a far, far better thing I do than I have ever done before.

Anyway, here I am, looking upwards and thinking that this is a far far worse thing that anything I've ever done before. Worse than my experience of knitting at school. Eventually someone notices me and seeing the cardboard box, directs me to the guillotine which is round the corner.

I pull up there in surprise. For a start, this gadget now before me doesn't look at all like the guillotine in the film. And the operator doesn't look like an executioner either because if I remember correctly, the one in the film hadn't been wearing a mini skirt and jumper and bright red lipstick. 'Are you here to have the box cut down to size?' this female executioner asks me quite pleasantly, a big smile on her face.

I can only nod, thinking that yet again my vivid imagination has been running riot. And even though I've really known from the start that my life has not been in danger and my job is assured, I am still very disappointed that the guillotine is not like the French one.

With a job and money and what with mixing with new people, I soon begin to grow more confident. And this new-found confidence even extends to my discovering where I can get a studio photograph taken to send to Mac. So on Saturday afternoon I iron my hair, almost doing a Van Gogh trick on my ear with the hot iron. But the end result when I look in the mirror is a Leonardo Di Vinci masterpiece.

In the studio, the photographer sets me up nicely, getting the pose right. And then just as the camera snaps, so does my bra strap. I only hope it isn't my own rubber that has let me down. A mysterious little smile that plays about my lips at the critical moment is captured by the camera. This clears up at long last, the enigma of the Mona Lisa's grin. It was all due to a snapping Playtex.

The weeks and months go by and when autumn comes it is hard to believe that I have been writing to Mac for almost a year. We write almost every day and by now know more about each other than we do about ourselves. Mac is into books in a big way and is always writing about the latest one he's read – half a dozen a week from the sound of it.

His favourite writer is Graham Greene, but he also sings the praises of Hemingway and someone called Alan Sillitoe and John McGahern and Joyce and Chekhov. When I see F. Scott Fitzgerald on the list I think that Mac doesn't like him and that the capital F. is shorthand for a swear word so I'm shocked.

But Celia puts me right and explains that the F stands for Francis and that if Mac likes all those writers, then he's obviously an intellectual like herself. She desperately wants to be thought of as an intellectual. She is always going on about existentialism and the proletariat and the bourgeoisie. But when I ask her to explain what they mean, she tells me that I wouldn't understand. If I want to learn I will have to start at the beginning with Plato. All I know about him is that he advocated Platonic friendships which involved 'no hands on experience at all'. I feel that's going a bit too far!

But I want to be an intellectual to impress Mac and so I agree to read Plato. And I try. I do really try. But when he starts going on about a chair being or not being in a room when I am or amn't there, it all becomes a bit too much. Particularly when I try it out.

I put a chair in the front room and warn everyone not to touch it while I am at work, ignoring the odd looks and mutterings. All day I can hardly wait to get home to see what might have happened. But when I do get home, the chair is there exactly as I left it (this is a bit unusual as nothing is ever left alone in our house). It is still sitting there in the evening and, disappointed that the experiment isn't working, I decide to place the chair in the hall when I go to bed. Again, I warn everyone not to touch it.

Later that night I am awoken by a crash from downstairs and what sounds to me like cursing and swearing. I wonder about the chair and if it is still safely in its place, but I am too frightened to go down and check.

The next morning, however, I am shaken to the core when I go downstairs and find that the chair has gone. I rush into the kitchen to pronounce to the world my latest and most significant finding, only to be confronted by my father demanding who'd put a bloody chair at the bottom of the stairs the previous night. He'd been out for a pint and had fallen over it when he came home.

I decide then that Plato is doubly dangerous. Not only can he ruin your love life but cripple your father as well. So I decide that there will be no more Plato for me. Bring on Elvis Presley instead. He might drive my father mad with his singing and gyrating, but so far he hasn't tried to cripple him.

So after all this, I decide not to mention my experiments to Mac. By this point we are madly in love – a love that depends solely on the postman. I'm sure the post office has no idea that they are almost solely responsible for keeping our love alive, even if merely platonically, or how important they are to both of us. I don't ever want to imagine what will happen if they go on strike, which seems to be the national disease at this time.

I rarely see the morning postman as I've already left for work by the time he calls. But the afternoon postman is almost a member of the family, I see him so often. Almost every day he sits out-side the factory with my letter. And if he is further down the road and I am on my way out of work, I know by the speed of the van that he has a letter for me.

The letters are to-ing and fro-ing at a great rate and without a hitch. What a great service! Never a letter lost. This is partly due to the efficiency of the post office and partly due to St Anthony. I always put S.A.G. on the back of all my letters. One day at work, a male colleague asks me what the letters mean.

'Saint Anthony Guide,' I tell him.

'What?'

'Saint Anthony Guide. It means that that letter won't get lost.'

'Don't be daft,' he derides me.

'Well it won't,' I say. 'That letter will arrive safely in London.'

'Why?' he demands. 'And who's this Saint Anthony fella any-way? The Chief Postmaster?' He is scathing.

A fat lot he knows about saints. Obviously a Protestant, I think. 'No,' I say now. 'Saint Anthony's the patron saint of lost things.'

'But the letter isn't lost.'

'Well, I'm only ensuring that he finds it in case it does get lost.'

'Huh,' he scoffs and walks away in total disbelief.

A week later, I discover that a strange thing has happened with that letter. I had forgotten to put the house number on the address. The house is on a very long street in bedsitter land in London. And to make matters worse, each house on the street contains four or five flats. In one of them lives Mac.

But some Cupid in the Post Office must have been informed by someone (Saint Anthony, as far as I'm concerned) who the let-ter is for because when Mac receives it, it has written on it in large letters: 'TRY 24', which is the number of the house he lives in. Now I gladly inform my colleague that Saint Anthony has indeed looked after my letter. But he is definitely a Protestant for he claims that it would have paid me better to have ensured I got the address right in the first place, and forgot all about the S.A.G.

In July I reach the ripe old age of 21, but there is no celebratory party to mark the occasion. Though officially an adult now, I still really have no sense. At heart I am still a teenager with the same attitudes I've had for years. While I know most women of my age might wish to be with a Hollywood hunk, I on the other hand still want to be like one. And Clint Eastwood is still my first choice.

I try to swagger like him which isn't easy with a limp and a pair of thirty eights in their Playtex holsters. But I have a natural narrowing of one eye from trying to cope with my short sightedness, so that's one small advantage. My thumbs are still always stuck in my jeans' pockets, ready for the draw and all that's missing is the cigar and the mule.

Mac promises do his Mae West bit at the end of the summer and come to visit me. But as the Olympic Games begin, he becomes ill with a blood-poisoned foot. So while athletes are breaking all kinds of records, running, hopping and jumping, and Olga Korbet is doing things no self-respecting Irish girl would ever do (even fully clothed), Mac is sitting in London with his feet up, ogling Olga no doubt.

He will come to visit me, he tells me, when the foot is better. So there is nothing for me to do but wait. If I'd had two good legs, I think, I could practise at being a gymnast and give Mac a surprise when he did come visiting, while wearing all my clothes of course. But it is Mac who has the surprise for me.

20

Into the West

∽

Towards the end of September, a letter arrives from Mac. After all this time, there can be no mistaking his handwriting on the envelope. Nor can I mistake the Irish stamp. Is St Anthony playing tricks I wonder? It's all I need right now – a saint who's a practical joker.

I feverishly and apprehensively tear open the envelope. When I look at the letter the first thing I notice is that the address is Mac's home address in the west. Trembling all over, I read on, not certain whether I can believe what I see. Mac is in Ireland – he's come without telling me, wishing to give me a surprise. And what's more, he's planning on coming to visit me the next day. This is no surprise. This is total shock – and for a variety of reasons.

First of all, I am not at all prepared for a meeting. I really need time to psyche myself up, whatever that means. I want to project the image of the perfect woman for him when he comes – a woman who is able to cook and clean and sew (I've already given up on the knitting and as I'm certainly not willing to consider 'vigorous' courting, I feel that I need some attributes that might impress him). All along I'd hoped that Mac would give me a couple of week's warning as to when he might arrive so that I could take a crash course in some of those womanly arts. But now I've got to get the hang of them all in less than 24 hours.

Though I am now getting on (21 seems ancient) I still have not mastered the domestic sciences. This, no doubt, is due to my having been too busy playing at being Clint Eastwood, who only ever seemed to eat beans and who simply cut a hole in a blanket when he wanted something to keep out the cold.

So how am I to face Mac, who has already informed me that, for the most part, he eats out? By now, no doubt, he is well used to the haute cuisine of London? His favourite eating place, he's told me, is the Wimpy. When I mentioned this to my brother, he told me that they are the largest construction company in England. So now I'm convinced that Mac must be very important to be eating out with them. I assume, of course, that he doesn't wear one of their donkey jackets or the yellow hat, while doing so.

As it happens, I don't have much time to dwell on these matters anyway. The letter arrives on Thursday afternoon and Mac arrives exactly 24 hours later. He has with him a box of chocolates and is wearing about his neck the biggest medallion I've ever seen, which looks, to all intents and purposes, both in weight and size, like the wheel rim of a bus. I've told him I like the hippie look but this looks more like Mark Spitz's seven gold medals smelted down and made into one. If he ever falls into water while wearing it, he'll sink like a stone.

But I think him to be very romantic. The medallion must be weighing him down, yet despite that he's still worn it and I know he's worn it just for me. I introduce him to the family, leave him with them in the sitting room and dash upstairs. I'm so nervous, I need time to pull myself together. Something has set my pulse racing and I wonder if it can be the size of that medallion.

I wonder too how this stranger will get on with my mad family who will certainly interrogate him once I've left the room. God only knows what they are going to make of the medallion. I feel terrible about leaving him there alone with them but I just have to have time to myself. But Mac turns out to be a diplomat, if nothing else. With me out of the way, he gives the chocolates to my mother and from that moment on she will not have a wrong word said against him.

Upstairs, I am a nervous wreck and I pace about, trying to think, trying to sort out how I am going to react in a sane and normal manner. I need to remain cool. Think Clint Eastwood, I urge myself. He wouldn't fall apart. So I square my shoulders, thrust my chest out – not too far – and pull myself together. I tidy my make up a bit more, hitch my gun belt on my hip and go out to meet my fate, like Dirty Harry.

Or rather, I return back downstairs. Mac is still there waiting for me, a big smile on his face. He's quite obviously survived the interrogation from my parents. In fact I think he's passed with honours. So we are now free to go out. I think they feel that he will be quite safe with me and will defend his virtue against anything I might throw at him.

We decide to go out alone, with no one with us but ourselves. I decide to boldly go where I have never gone before, up the Windy Gap into the Clare Hills. Well, Mac has a car, so we're free to do so.

But there is one little matter which must be taken care of before we can be alone. Celia wants a lift into the city centre and naturally, being the gentleman he is, Mac obliges. The three of us set off to walk from our front door to the main road where Mac has parked his car. The footpath is only wide enough for two abreast and Mac walks in front. We walk behind like any true unliberated woman. 'Where's the car?' my sister calls out to him.

'Just up here,' he says proudly.

We look up but we can only see one car parked on the road. 'Is that it?' Celia asks pointing to the black Morris Minor.

'Yes,' he proclaims, prouder still I think.

We both giggle, but I don't think Mac gets the joke.

Despite my misgivings, I discover that you can wine and dine her in an old Morris Minor, even without the food or the drink. Yet despite this, there is one hiccup. It's too dark to find the Windy Gap. So we do the next best thing and drive to some other gap where we park and look down on the lights of the city far below.

Here, all alone on top of the hill, we sit and talk and talk and it seems as though we have known each other all our lives. He has a present for me – a silver heart-shaped locket. As I take it and see its pale and silvery form in the palm of my hand, I just can't believe that this guy here beside me actually loves me.

I feel a need for honesty and truthfulness coming on. I have learned the skill of pushing everything that is good away from me before it gets too good and I am once more disappointed. And so I do what surely no woman on a first date has ever done before. It is a truly odd thing to do, though I don't exactly see it that way.

So I ask Mac the big question. 'Do you want to see my leg?'

What can he say but yes, even if his voice sounds a little shaky and croaky?

And so I roll up my jeans to the knee on the left leg, remove my sneaker and ankle sock, and show him the scars and the mis-shapen foot. Then I show him the blue-tinged leg that is always cold to the touch. I do not show him the other leg. He looks at it in the dark quite disinterestedly I think, and merely goes, 'Hmmm.'

I don't know how I feel. I don't know what I want to hear. But he says nothing, only puts his arm about my shoulders and pulls my head down onto his chest. The sharp edges of that damn great medallion cut into my cheek but I don't care. I could stay like this forever. And as we sit in the dark and cuddle, I know that this guy really does not care a jot about my bad leg. He can't see it. He can only see ME.

I am in heaven as we return home later that night, a relieved Mac with his virtue still intact – only just though. All the family are up and waiting for us and seem happy that we're both home safely. While we've been out, they've laid into the chocolates. But I don't care and I am only too happy to take one when my sister proffers me the now sadly depleted box.

The next day, I try to impress Mac with my culinary skills. 'A man's heart is in his stomach,' I'd always been told. So I think it's a good idea to show my man that I can cook (even though I can't) and that his stomach at least will be in good hands.

I decide on lamb cutlets. After all, what can go wrong with them? Well, one could forget that they were frying in the pan for a start. And being an expert at making a mess of things, I do just that. I forget all about them and they are burned to a frazzle. But he is so in love that he just doesn't care. He even bravely tries to eat them and when I slip out of the kitchen, red with embarrassment, I can hear him crunching and grinding away. He does make a great heroic effort to eat as much as possible and I'm really glad that I now know his heart, if not exactly in his stomach, is still in the right place.

I have to go to work the next day but I've arranged to take a half day and plan to go on a picnic in the afternoon. But when I get home, there is no sign of the love of my life. He has already gone out and I am bitterly disappointed. I'm told that my father has taken him off to show him the sights and delights of Limerick.

I certainly wouldn't have known my way around the city anyway so if he wanted a guided tour of the Walls of Limerick, Patrick Sarsfield's statue, the Treaty Stone and King John's Castle, he would have found me sadly inadequate as a guide. He would have also discovered that I didn't know where all the pubs in Limerick were either. But my father is an expert guide in that area too and keeps Mac, who happens to be a strict teetotaller, out for most of the day.

When they return, my father merry from all the porter no doubt Mac has bought him, and Mac himself with a sad dog look on his face at missing me, I can't stay mad for long. Anyway, I understand that Mac could not very well leave my father in one of the pubs and come back home alone, though as he has a passionate dislike of pubs, I do know that that is what he would have liked to do.

The next day Mac takes me off to Mayo to meet his family. It is a long drive in the Morris Minor and a great adventure for me. I think that it is on this drive that I find that I have a great love for travelling. I love the new scenes and the towns we pass through that up to now were only names on a map. The sheer unbridled pleasure of being all alone with Mac, who talks and sings non stop, is simply wonderful.

Eventually we reach Mayo. I have only been to Mayo on the few occasions that I've come to Knock as a child. It seems strange to pass through Knock where I had come so many years ago, seeking a miracle. Now that I am back here, I feel that at last I've got my miracle. I have found true love and what else can matter?

I have never really got to know any western people – apart from the cowboys – and so I am very shy at meeting Mac's family for a great many reasons, and am both glad and relieved when the initial introductions are over. They appear to be pleasant, warm and welcoming people, and they make me feel right at home. I can see where Mac gets his attributes from.

But there is one member of the family, a sister, who is not at home, and Mac asks his mother where she is. 'She's back the mountain getting the cows,' his mother replies.

I'm horrified. I think of poor old St Patrick, who had been all alone up there on Slieve Mish, minding all those sheep. But that was in 432 and this is 1972. And further more, this is a young girl they're referring to. Surely what she's doing is deadly dangerous. What if she falls off the mountain?

Terrible visions of Mount Everest with cows and a young girl all alone on its summit, swirl through my head. Mountain climbing with a good team of climbers and sherpas (whatever they are) is one thing, I think. But climbing with cows? It doesn't bear thinking about. So naturally I am very worried.

'How do the cows get up the mountain?' I ask Mac when I have some time alone with him.

'We drive them up there,' he answers, cool as you like and as if it is the most natural thing in the world.

'In a lorry?' I ask.

'A lorry?' He looks askance at me. 'Where would we get a lorry? We just drive them up. You know, walk behind them and drive them along.'

I still can't picture cows walking up a mountain but I let that go for the moment. 'Why do you drive them up there?' I ask.

'To graze,' he says, laughing at the city girl's ignorance.

'And then ye bring them back down again?'

'Well, yes, of course. They have to be brought down for milking.'

'But isn't that very dangerous?' I persist.

'Not at all,' he scoffs. 'We do it every day.'

I am confused. These people in the west of Ireland seem very strange to say the least. No one else is a bit worried about this young girl, but I am and I can't relax until she arrives home safely with the cows. And then when she breezes in, she doesn't seem a bit worried about her experience.

'What would you like to do while you're here?' Mac asks me later.

I have never really been anywhere before that I can remember except to Knock and to Croom. I have never seen mountains – at least not close up, and certainly not ones with cows on the top.

'I'd love to go and see the mountain,' I say, 'if that's OK with you?'

'Sure,' he says. 'We'll go tomorrow morning after breakfast.'

The next morning I am really looking forward to seeing the mountain. I've visions of a beautiful blue and purple mountain with a river flowing at the bottom. Being a cowboy at heart, I've always been fascinated by mountains and this will be my first time seeing a real one close up.

I'm feeling terribly excited as we set off. It isn't too far, Mac says. He knows I'm not able to walk terribly far, especially on rough terrain. We walk and walk but I cannot see a trace of a mountain at all. Perhaps it's down in a hollow, I think. Eventually we arrive at some very heathery looking land which is virtually flat except for a few bumps and humps here and there. 'Well, this is it,' Mac says.

'Where?' I know my eyes aren't great but they aren't that bad either and they would hardly miss a great big mountain. I know it's not Mount Everest I'm going to see – in fact, I accept that this mountain probably doesn't even have a name – but even Mohammed wouldn't be fooled by what's before me. There's simply nothing to see.

'Here,' Mac says. 'This land all about here is the mountain.' He waves his hand to take in all this brown flat terrain.

I can't help it. I roar out laughing. 'That's not a mountain.' Now it's my turn to scoff. 'A mountain is a great big tall yolk going thousands of feet up into the sky.'

'Ah,' he says. 'You're obviously thinking of a big mountain. Well, we don't have any of those around here.'

It seems to me that they don't have any small mountains either but I don't say so. I think the people in the west are very strange indeed. Even their mountains lie flat on the ground.

I look disappointed so Mac explains they describe this piece of bog and heather as mountainy land – ergo the mountain for short. And as he knows I'm bitterly disappointed, he asks me if he can make it up to me.

'OK,' I say. 'You can take me to see Croke Park.'

'Croke Park!' He's obviously astonished. 'You never said you were interested in football. Anyway, I don't know if there's any match on there just now.'

Now it's my turn to be astonished. And I wonder if Mac is losing it. How can he imagine that you could play football on top of a mountain. I'd seen pictures of Croke Park and there seemed to be hardly any room on the top of it, barely enough I'd say for St Patrick to lie down while he was up there.

The poor old saint obviously didn't learn his lesson on Slieve Mish, for as soon as he came back to Ireland and got to Mayo, there he was haring up the mountain named after him like a billy goat. And not only that, but then didn't he stay up there for 40 days and 40 nights. Well, I only want to see this mountain. I don't want to climb it – not that I could with my bad leg – never mind stay up there alone.

Mac eventually realises what I mean and laughs. 'You mean Croagh Patrick,' he says. 'Croke Park is where they play football and hurling.'

We have a good laugh about that and then Mac points out Croagh Patrick to me. It is like a small faint triangle in the far distance, blending into the background of pale blue sky. He promises to take me there on my next visit to Mayo and assures me that, despite looking so small, it is a proper mountain.

The few days we have together pass all too quickly and then it is time for Mac to return to London. We can't bear to be parted so I go with him on the train to Dublin and we just sit together in each other's arms, wishing that time would stand still. But it doesn't and the long train journey is over much too quickly.

Our time at the station is very short. Mac has to hurry to catch the train which will take him to the boat and then I am left alone. I feel so lost and lonely that I want to run after him and go off with him. But I can't. I will just have to bear the loneliness until we meet again. We promise to meet at Christmas. I will go to London. Me, who would go nowhere alone, is now planning to travel to London.

I stay with a friend in Dublin and travel home alone to Limerick on the train the next day. Here I throw myself into my work to kill the ache of loneliness. Were the golf balls better or worse in 1972? Did underwear elastic get tighter or looser? How they fared depended, I think, on how I was feeling each day – elated and sad and happy all at the same time and longing for Christmas, as I'd never longed for it as a child.

21

ON CLOUD NINE

❀

December comes round and I am going off to London to be with Mac again, and have a holiday. At last I will get a glimpse of the great big world that is out there and that I now want to see and explore. And here I am too, about to fly for the very first time. It is both exciting and terrifying.

When I get to the airport and board the plane I'm frightened by this huge mechanical bird. I can't understand how something so big can fly, with all those people in it and all their luggage as well. I had once tried jumping off a high wall with an umbrella held open above my head, believing that I would soar away through the sky like Mary Poppins. But while I did feel some resistance, I still came down to earth with a bang. And it would appear to me that the laws of physics are pretty simple and straightforward. If you're heavier than air, then down you come.

So you can imagine my terror when I board the plane which certainly is heavier than air. I find a seat (well I don't really find it; it has been there all the time) I sit down and fasten my seat belt, rigid in my seat. I don't really need the belt. I am much too scared to move. The plane is already two hours late taking off and by the look of things will be later still.

I look out the window at the tarmac to take my mind off things. I try to open the window but it won't budge. This is a bit worrying as I feel I need air. And as I know that there is less oxygen the higher up you go, I feel that I will certainly need fresh air when we're high in the sky. Perhaps then some of the other passengers will open their windows and I'll be all right.

The plane now makes a roaring noise and we begin to move. It's a bit bumpy but the ride doesn't last too long. Then suddenly it makes an even more terrible roaring noise and shoots forwards, all but pinning me back in my seat. I clench my eyes tight shut and say a prayer to St Christopher, honorary Chairman of Aer Lingus.

And then just as suddenly the plane stops. When I open my eyes, I notice now that the cabin is tilted upwards and I wonder if we've got a front wheel puncture and they've jacked up the plane to change the tyre. But I think they should have told us this at the very least. Now we're going to be even later. Anyway, it levels out again (the tyre must be changed) and I sit and wait and wait for something to happen. But the plane just stands still.

I look out the window but all that's out there is a grey fog which seems to have come down very quickly. I realise that planes can't fly in the fog so we're obviously waiting for it to clear. Only if it doesn't clear I'll never get to London.

The hostesses now give us something to eat. I watch in amazement as these girls walk up and down the plane with tea and coffee. Some of the passengers even have the nerve to walk about too. They go through a door at the top, obviously getting off to stretch their legs. I hope the captain doesn't decide to take off suddenly and leave them behind.

By now I am getting really worried. Mac is to meet me off the plane at Heathrow. But I am now hours late and surely he will think that I'm not coming and go home. Well, it's what I would do. I wish the plane would just go. Now I wouldn't even be scared of flying, I'm so anxious to be up in the sky. What is keeping this plane from taking off? It has to be the fog but I can't understand why they haven't explained this. I'd love to ask the hostesses or even one of the other passengers about the delay but I'm much too shy.

And then, just while all this is going through my mind, the captain's voice comes over the loudspeaker announcing that we will be landing in London in ten minutes. I can't believe it. We haven't even taken off yet, it's at least an hour to Heathrow and here's this man, who's in charge of the plane if you don't mind, claiming that he can make it there in ten minutes. What a boaster! But then I think that maybe I'm on Concorde and that explains it.

When I look out the window I notice that the grey has disappeared and there is what looks like blue sky flying past the window (I'm not fooled though. I remember that first train journey and the platform moving away while the train stayed still. So we're moving through the sky).

The realisation dawns on me that we are up in the sky and I freeze. Slowly I lean over to look out the window. Below me I can see houses and green fields and trees and cars. I'm actually up in the sky, in a plane, and there's no rope or chain holding us up. The captain's made a fool of us all. He's pretended that we're on the ground all the time while we're actually in the sky.

Thankfully I don't have much time to dwell on this fact because before I know it, we have landed safely and everyone begins to stand up. I try in vain to open my seat belt, but it won't budge. I'm trapped. I keep pulling and pulling but it's no use. I'm stuck here and the plane will probably take off again in a minute and I'll end up back in Shannon or even worse, in New York, where the plane originally came from.

People begin to remove their luggage from the overhead storage compartments and to disembark. As the plane empties, I am still stuck in my seat. Panic is setting in as if I wasn't panicking enough already. I have a vision now of being a stowaway, ending up in Timbuktu and being carted off to jail.

At last a real gentleman, standing in the aisle, notices my agitation and predicament and asks if I need some help. 'I can't seem to undo my seat belt,' I say helplessly.

'Allow me,' he says gallantly. It's the highlight of the flight – the damsel in distress being rescued by her knight in shining –

well blue pinstripe – armour. He pulls back the silver buckle clip, undoes the belt and I am free and feeling rather silly. But there are no instructions on the belt and I'm a woman who lives by instructions.

Now I still have to find my man. But first I have to find my luggage. I think the captain will be outside the plane handing out the luggage. But there's no sign of him. And there's no sign of Mac either. I just knew it. He's gone home. As I look around, completely lost and bewildered, a couple take pity on me and befriend me. They tell me to come with them and they'll help me get my luggage and wait with me until I find Mac. Or what's more than likely, he finds me.

It's just as well they take me under their wing for I wouldn't know what to do or where to go. I know nothing about carousels, but eventually me and my luggage are reunited. The airport is very busy and I don't think I've ever before seen so many people in one place.

Or that's what I think until my saviours take me out into the Arrivals' Hall. Here there are simply millions of people milling about and there seems to be total chaos. You just might spot the tallest man on earth here, but certainly not Mac, who stands five feet nothing in his stockings. How I wish I'd sent him that booklet from the height specialist. At least he might have got elongated arms and he could have stuck one of them up in the air and waved it about to attract my attention.

I am lost. I look lost. I feel lost. Mac will never find me and what will become of me then? I am terror stricken. But the couple who've taken me under their wing are either seasoned travellers, or intelligent, or have a bit of common sense, and they tell me not to worry. They will have Mac paged at the main desk and we'll find him that way.

Yet just as the announcement is being made, there is Mac miraculously beside me. Realising that he would never find me in the crowd, he too had come to the main desk to have me paged and just found me waiting there for him. Everything is wonderful and I am floating on air as Mac and I greet each other shyly, just like two love-lost teenagers, which in a way is what we are, despite being the ripe old age of 21.

When I realise that Mac has a great deal of intelligence and common sense, having had the initiative to page me, I know I'm in good solid hands. I need love but I need someone to take care of me too. And I know in that moment that I've found my man. Despite being no higher than Clint Eastwood's knee, I know that Mac will never allow anyone to laugh at me or mock me or hurt me ever again. I'll be safe from now on from the slings and arrows of the world and from the sticks and stones too.

London is wonderful and Mac shows it all to me. He has a car fitted with an eight track stereo cassette player, and to the sounds of Simon and Garfunkel, Rod Stewart and Leonard Cohen, he shows me the sights. I can't see any tapes of Johnny Cash about and I realise he must have hidden them. Johnny Cash had featured strongly in that first tape Mac had sent me the previous Christmas and I hadn't been too enthusiastic about him.

But even continuous Johnny Cash songs couldn't dampen my excitement and pleasure now as Mac shows me the lights of Regent Street. And yes, they are simply breathtaking. As I stand in Trafalgar Square beneath Nelson's Column (he still hasn't jumped) pigeons come and perch on my outstretched arms. When one perches on my shoulder, I really feel at last that I am Short Joan Silver and I never want to be anyone else again. While the gigantic Christmas tree, festooned with what seems to be millions of brightly-coloured lights, gleams and glints and dazzles me, it is little wonder that I think I'm dreaming.

The only disappointment is Piccadilly Circus. There's no big top, no clowns or lions or tigers – not even a rope to fall over. But then there is the Tower of London and Buckingham Palace to make up for it; and Chelsea Bridge at night with the lights swirling on the water of the Thames. Now, here at last, is my river.

We drive down the King's Road where all the pop stars go and I see the British Museum where Mac spends his Sunday afternoons, gazing at the manuscripts and dreaming of one day being a writer and having his books in the library there. Because it's Christmas, all the tourist attractions are closed, but just seeing them from the outside is a magical experience. This is the greatest city in the world, Mac tells me, and I'm amazed and proud that this young man from the mountain in Mayo knows his way around and can drive in the traffic which seems endless. And loves me, bad leg and all.

The night following St Stephen's Day (they call it Boxing Day here I learn) Mac takes me up to the top of the hill on which Alexandra Palace stands and shows me the view. I can't believe a city can be so big. It is so much bigger than Limerick. The lights, spread out before us, seem to go on and on forever.

In the magic of the endless lights, Mac speaks, and what comes from his lips sounds very much like a proposal of marriage. As these have been scarce in my life, and if the past is anything to go by, could prove scarce in the future, I decide not to take any chances. Yes, I say, yes with some of the enthusiasm of Molly Bloom, if not exactly with her accompanying activities. Best get that yes in, I think, before Mac can change his mind.

And then, just for assurance's sake, I ask him for an engagement ring. I don't know if Mac equates a proposal with an engagement, but in true honourable round table fashion, he promises to take me to the jewellers the very next day and buy me the most beautiful, the most gorgeous ring – the best darn engagement ring in the place – with one proviso. It must be really cheap. It's a sign of the intimacy we share that we can talk like this. After all, what other girl on being promised an engagement ring would have to also accept that it had to be a really cheap one?

We go out the next day to Wood Green High Road and there in Zale's Jeweller's he buys me the ring. It has one diamond in a diamond-shaped setting, which you might just be able to see with an electronic microscope if your eyesight was good. And it isn't the cheapest ring in the shop either, even if only just. It's mine and I'm engaged to be married. I can see it glistening and glittering and I would be willing to swear that only the Koohinoor Diamond is bigger – and then only just.

Mac takes me out to celebrate this momentous purchase and this momentous occasion, no, not with a candlelit dinner for two with a gypsy playing love songs for us on a violin. Instead we go to the cinema to see Disney's *Snow White and the Seven Dwarfs*. The dwarfs are probably bigger than the two of us, but they don't get engaged or get to buy Snow White a diamond ring, or don't, as Mac rudely points out, get to have a fling with her either.

Time passes in fleeting moments of great happiness and then my holiday is over and I have to go back home. I don't realise as I fly out of Heathrow Airport that in a few short months London is going to be my home.

I am heartbroken at leaving Mac, who is just as devastated, but yet I'm also on Cloud Nine again at the thought that I'm engaged to be married. I am so looking forward to surprising my mother, that I can hardly wait to get home.

'Well how did you enjoy your holiday?' my mother asks

'Great,' I say. 'London is the most wonderful place I've ever seen. And by the way, Mam, do you like my ring?' I ask, proudly showing off my left hand, where I hope the diamond is glittering.

'It's nice,' she says. 'But what kind of ring is it?'

'It's an engagement ring.'

'A what?'

'An engagement ring,' I repeat.

'But sure you don't know that fellow at all,' she says.

'Of course I do,' I protest.

'But sure you only know him for a few weeks.'

'But I've been writing to him for over a year.'

Our local Parish Priest happens to be visiting that day and my mother turns to him for moral support. 'Now, what do you think of her, Father,' she says, 'to go over there to London and come back engaged to a fellow she hardly knows?'

But I get my spoke in before he can reply. 'Wouldn't you know someone better, Father,' I say, 'by writing to them, rather than meeting them in person?'

The priest, bless him, agrees and I think that is good enough for my mother. She accepts the inevitable in her own way and I think that secretly she's probably glad and maybe relieved that I'm going to have someone of my own to take care of me in the future when she's no longer around to do so. And I think too her head has been turned a little by that box of chocolates.

The new year moves on and the days pass in a blur of pining for Mac and waiting for his letters, counting seconds and minutes and hours until I see him again. I am so in love, so full of life, that my mother doesn't know what to do with me. I am in great form – no more moods, no more fights, no more aggro. I'm just happy and silly and witty. My mother's wonderful phrase for falling in love is, 'You got a slap of the saucepan', and now she constantly says to me, 'When you got a slap of the saucepan, you got a right slap of the saucepan'. And I did. But I will get my own back on the saucepans in due time.

The wedding is set for September of that year. Mac is hoping to get a transfer to Ireland to work for a subsidiary of the company he presently works for as a service engineer, and this is supposed to happen in April. It's four months away and seems an eternity but somehow I'll manage to hang on.

And then disaster strikes. The recession in Ireland is biting hard and there is to be no transfer for Mac. If he stays on in London his job is secure as he's a highly-prized member of the firm's workforce there. If he comes to Ireland there will be no job for him here with the company's subsidiary, and he will find it difficult to find a job in another company. There are so few jobs, not even one for prized engineers like him.

He phones me one evening to tell me the bad news. We have no phone so we've arranged for Mac to call me each weekend at the public phone at the top of our housing estate. I have to go and wait there and hope that Mac is able to get a public phone on his side. This night I wait ages in the cold, and when no call is forthcoming, I decide to go home, bitterly disappointed that I can't hear his voice telling me he loves me.

I am almost home when I hear the phone ringing and then I have to run all the way back up to find that someone else has picked it up. But they very kindly give it to me when they realise it's for me. I am out of breath and Mac immediately wants to know if I am missing him that badly. I'm so glad to hear his voice that I can't be mad at him.

And then comes the bad news. There is not going to be a transfer. So now what do we do? Mac asks me to come to London – at least we will be together – but as I am not willing to live in sin with him – that means I would have to live in a flat on my own. And I just know that I would be too terrified to live alone in London. It was magical at Christmas but living alone there – now that's a different matter.

'So what shall we do then?' Mac asks. 'I don't want to be alone for much longer. I miss you too much.'

'Well, we could get married,' I say.

'When?' he asks, as if this suggestion is the most natural in the world. Obviously he hasn't got cold feet or changed his mind.

I pause while I do some quick calculations in my head. I find I am still good at maths. 'How about in three weeks time, that's the Saturday after Easter?' I suggest.

'OK,' he says. Just like that. It would appear that I'm not the only one who's been clobbered with the saucepan.

And so it is decided just like that, as Tommy Cooper might say. Indeed if it hadn't been for it being Lent, a time when one cannot get married, I might have set the date even earlier.

When I tell my parents what we've decided, they go into shock. But it's nothing compared to the shock the same old Parish Priest gets when I go to see him and tell him I want to get married.

'When?' he asks.

'In three week's time, Father.'

'Oh, but that's impossible,' he says

'Oh, but I have to get married, Father,' I tell him. After he has recovered a little from this shock, I explain the situation to him. He is very understanding about it all and tells me he will do his best for us. But firstly, of course, I will need to obtain my parents' consent.

'But I'm over 21, Father,' I say. And so I am, but with all the common sense I display, is it little wonder he thinks I'm still a teenager?

During the next few weeks I keep working and try making the arrangements for the wedding as well. I get great help from my father, who sorts out my birth certificate and letter of freedom. Then on 21 April Mac arrives home and comes to Limerick. It's great to have him with me again and now that he's here, I just know I'm doing the right thing. What's more heartening is that he thinks so too.

A few days later we have the rehearsal for the wedding and the priest comes to the house to go through the procedure. But because there is no privacy in our sitting room we use one of the bedrooms upstairs.

When the rehearsal is over and we have made our vows, I ask the priest, who is a very quiet shy man, 'Is that it Father?'

'Yes,' he says. 'That's it.'

'We're married then,' I say. 'So now we can hop into bed.'

'Oh no,' he says, mortified. 'You're not really married.'

'But you've just married us,' I say. 'We've just made our vows. And you did say that was it.'

The poor man is in a state. He doesn't seem to know what to do. 'Ah,' he says at last, 'you can't be married. There were no witnesses, do you see.'

I laugh and he realises that I was only joking. If he only knew, there was no way I was going to miss my big day.

22

SOMETHING OLD, SOMETHING NEW

❧

The day before the wedding arrives. I have no nerves and work right up until lunch time. Then it is a sad farewell to my colleagues and the end of another phase in my life.

After lunch I visit my Great Uncle in hospital, the same one where I was once tied to a cot and I once worked. It seems as if it will always play a part in my life. My uncle is dying and I know I will never see him again.

When I leave the hospital I go into the city centre. I have arranged to meet Celia at 3pm outside her place of work. I'm a little early so I take the long way round to the factory and here I wait outside the entrance. And I wait and wait. I am very patient and stand there for a whole half hour. Still being terribly shy, I'm too scared to go into the factory and see what's happened.

But eventually I realise that I have to do something and I muster up as much courage as I can. I bravely go where I normally wouldn't venture, only to be informed that Celia left ages ago.

When I hear this I become furious. How could she do this to me, today of all days? She must know that the shops will be closing at 5.30pm and I have so much to do and so little time in which to do it.

I clamp down on my fury and weigh things up in my mind. It is much too late to go home and get someone else to help me.

And I cannot do everything that has to be done on my own. Oh, to heck with it all, I think. It is hopeless. I won't bother getting married in the morning.

I storm off, not certain of my direction, and my old faithful, left leg, chooses this moment to let me down. I fall flat on the pavement and graze my hands and knees. I am even more upset now, not to mention being mortally embarrassed.

As I pick myself up, I see Celia. My whole future, I realise, my whole life, depends on the next few minutes. I can give out to her and then she'll retaliate, and that will be that. Or I can remain cool and calm. I decide on the latter course of action. Oh, where, oh, where is the Valium when you most need it? With all the self control I can muster up, I say, 'What happened to you?'

'I got out early so we would have more time,' she says, calm as you like. 'What happened to you?'

'I was too early so I took the long way round. I've been up at the factory waiting for you for the past half hour. Anyway, I suppose we had best do what we have to do.' I speak quietly, calmly and reasonably, but inside I'm fuming.

Our first job is to collect the three-tier wedding cake from the bakery and take it to the hotel. It is much heavier than we anticipate. Celia takes the two smaller tiers and I take the large bottom one. So here we are, staggering up O'Connell Street, carrying three tiers of wedding cake and resting the boxes on every second car bonnet. By the time we get halfway up the street, we're wrecked. Marathon running will be nothing to us after this.

But now a major obstacle faces us. We have to cross the street. There are no traffic lights here and no pedestrian crossing – not even a zebra escaped from the circus. And I have never seen so wide a street or one so daunting to cross as O'Connell Street this day. It has certainly become twice as wide since I last saw it. I wish that there were some nice irresponsible drivers about who might have parked their cars across the street so as to assist me in carrying my wedding cake. But all the cars – and there seems to be millions of them, not to mention buses and lorries - are continuously whizzing by at hundreds of miles per hour.

'We'll never make it across,' I say to Celia.

'We will,' she says confidently. Much too confidently for my liking. 'Just take a deep breath and run for it.'

Run! We've barely been crawling along, carrying the cake from car to car and I'm already exhausted. I don't even have the energy to take a deep breath and for once my extra large lungs are redundant. At this rate, I'm not going to be a very energetic bride. In fact if I've got my breath back by the next day, it will be a miracle, though there's the consolation that Mac will almost certainly be thrilled with my heavy breathing.

Celia keeps on encouraging me. 'You have to try,' she says. 'It's not that far.'

Well, only half a mile or so, I think. But then she has two tiers to carry and I've only got one. And being as it's my wedding this cake is meant to celebrate, I really should be the one with all the enthusiasm and energy. But when I think about crossing the street, my imagination runs riot.

It just won't go right. I know I will fall. I know I will. Then there will be cars screeching to a halt and Limerick will come to a standstill. And I will be sprawled prone in the middle of O'Connell Street with my face buried in my own wedding cake. That doesn't bear thinking about.

'Are you ready?' Celia asks.

I nod. What else can I do? And I tell myself that I am the one who jumped off the Hockey Wall. Now all I have to do is behave as I did that time – stupidly.

'Right,' Celia says. 'We'll go.'

With one tremendous burst of energy, we take off running, weighed down with three tiers of wedding cake. It seems an unending journey to the other pavement, but we make it, puffed and exhausted and jubilant. But we're not there yet.

We trek on up the side street to the hotel. Here, some idiot of an architect has put steps up to the entrance. There are five of them and they may as well be the pyramids of Egypt. I can't climb them.

Devastated, I stand looking at them, hating them, knowing that I cannot climb those steps carrying my tier of cake. I always need one hand to hold onto the banister when I climb the stairs. It will be impossible for me to carry the cake with one hand and hold the rail with the other. 'We'll make it,' Celia gasps when she sees the look of terror and resignation on my face.

'You might,' I puff. 'But I can't do it.'

The steps represent my Mount Everest at that moment and my strength is almost gone. I am hunched, exhausted over the cake. I can't go on. Sherpa Tensing in this situation would resign himself to failure, even if the Abominable Snowman was after him.

'Don't ever rest when you're exhausted,' Celia advises me now. 'Especially when you've only got a little bit more to go. It's much easier just to keep on going.'

Well, it might be if the mountain before me was the one Mac showed me when we were in Mayo. But this mountain before me is the real thing. I have to climb it and as I contemplate it, I hope that the guests will enjoy the cake tomorrow.

'We're almost there,' Celia coaxes. 'Just those few steps and we're there. Come on, you can do it.'

And so with all the strength I possess, I make a final supreme effort. All those years in the national school climbing the stairs without holding onto the banister come to my aid now. I sort of lean against the steel railing on the steps for support and, closing my eyes, somehow manage to climb this Everest. I don't know how I manage it but I do know it will go down as one of my greatest achievements.

Our remaining strength takes us through the door into the hotel. Here we plonk the three tiers on the reception desk and then fall against it, gasping for what might be our last breaths in this world, while the receptionist stares at us in astonishment. 'That's a wedding cake you've got there,' she says. 'Well, you can't leave it here.'

I now know why God has made this task of conveying my

wedding cake from the bakery to the hotel so difficult and exhausting. It's so that I don't have the energy when I get here to murder the receptionist. All I can do is gaze at her as if in a trance and gasp out the one word, 'What?'

'Wedding cakes cannot be left in the hotel during the day,' she explains. 'They can only be handed in at night after the hotel has closed or else brought to the hotel on the day of the wedding and then only just before the reception. The hotel cannot be held responsible for any wedding cakes left here during the day.'

I am still gasping and ready to burst into tears. 'Isn't there anything you can do?' I plead. 'We have just carried that cake all the way up O'Connell Street. We have faced death by misadventure and lack of air and exhaustion. I just can't face taking it away again. Right now, I'd be more willing to eat it, rather than do that.' She must think I'm serious for her face softens. 'Well maybe I could keep it here under the counter for you,' she says. 'But it will be at your own risk.'

I agree readily. No matter what the consequences, even if the cake disappears and we have to make do with a sponge cake, I couldn't bear to take that cake back down the street.

One job accomplished and time is getting on. Celia, who is to be my bridesmaid, now decides that it might be a good time to look for shoes. Of course, she has to look at every shoe in every shoe shop in Limerick. Finally, she decides on a pair and I drag her out of the shop in case she changes her mind.

I still have the flowers to pick up but now things begin to fall into place, and for a change, I'm not one of those things. The flowers are actually ready and waiting and don't weigh a ton like the cake. But the lady in the shop is determined to take every penny I have in return, it seems, for every flower in her shop. So I buy flowers for the lapels. This little bouquet would be perfect for my mother. And then, of course, the groom's mother will have to have one as well. I think the only one she doesn't suggest getting flowers for is the priest. And as I'm so confused, I'm not so sure even of that.

Maybe my common sense has escaped out the door, or this woman is the best sales woman in the world and can spot an easy target at a hundred paces, but she actually tries to sell me confetti. For my own wedding! And I actually buy it! But maybe that comes from a deep rooted knowledge that I have to be independent and do most things for myself.

We've everything done at last and then it's back home, worn out after carrying that damn cake. And now I have plenty of time to worry about whether or not the cake will still be there tomorrow. It should be the least of my worries, but after all that effort, I'd really be most disappointed with a sponge, even it was three tiered.

***

The next day dawns fine and cold but sunny. This is supposed to be the happiest day of my life. I decide that it should be just that. Stay calm is my motto and hope that Mac doesn't get cold feet. It's unlikely that he will, but I suppose it's every bride's fear.

The wedding ceremony itself is pretty conventional. I am dressed all in white, somewhere something blue is hidden away out of sight, but it's the pink flowers on my veil that upsets my mother. I should be all in white according to her, but I feel white enough as it is.

The music I've chosen for my walk up the aisle is the hymn 'How Great Thou Art' which is a big hit at this time (later Mac will tell me how delighted and honoured he is that I should have chosen that hymn. He thinks it refers to him). But it seems appropriate to me – God has to be great to have brought me to such a happy moment as this. And anyway I don't like *The Wedding March*. I've always thought it vulgar because of the way we sang it as children. Those self-same words go through my mind whenever I hear it played. It's certainly not very complimentary to any bride who is walking demurely up the aisle.

Here comes the bride,
All dressed in white,
With forty yards of elastic.
To keep her knickers tight.

I'm not having that. I don't want anyone singing those words under their breath while I'm walking past.

Now I am determined that I won't be late – I'm giving Mac no chance to get cold feet in the church – and so I arrive five minutes before noon, which is the time set for the great event to take place. As my wedding car, a local taxi festooned with ribbons, is about to pull into the church car park, a car races past at what must be 100 miles per hour, pulls in front of us with tyres screeching, and enters the car park. It's Mac and his brother who is to be his best man. By mere seconds, he's just managed not to be the first man in the world to turn up for his wedding later than his bride.

I watch in amazement as they both leap from the car and race for the church door, not daring to look back. Mac knows I'm superstitious and that the groom is not supposed to see his bride on their wedding day until she arrives at the altar (I knew all that letter writing would not go to waste and this, among many other things, is what we've discussed in the letters. Now, if we'd been together during all that time I don't think it's superstitions we'd have been talking about. That is, if we'd been talking at all).

Anyway, here's the groom and best man, the guests are here, the bride and her father are ready to make the long walk – and the priest is late. But he arrives, assuming that the bride will be late, and is embarrassed. Then the music begins and I'm ready to march, even if to a different tune.

The music is wonderful. I stand with my father in the church porch, listening and waiting for the point in the song where I will begin my walk. After a minute or so, the sacristan starts waving frantically at me to come on up to the altar. But I don't want to budge. It isn't time yet. I try to ignore her, but she is getting more frantic by the second.

I try to delay but my father is now telling me I have to go. It is still too early though – my whole timing will be ruined. I have planned to reach the top of the aisle as the song ends on what is a very high note. Now it will be a mess. And it's beginning to get very embarrassing indeed. The sacristan is heading down the aisle towards me, intent, it seems, on dragging me up to the altar. She must think I've got cold feet, or perhaps Mac has bribed her into dragging me up to the altar if I show any signs of reluctance.

I start walking. The sacristan is well down the church. I can see her hesitating. What does she do now? Does she keep on coming, does she duck into one of the seats or does she retreat? She chooses the latter and scurries back up towards the altar, crouching down like someone attacking the beaches at Normandy on D-day. I stifle a smile and am grateful for the loud music. It hides all the titters of amusement which are flitting about among the guests.

I walk very slowly, even by my standards, but the song is still ringing out when I reach the top seat. When I get to the spot where Mac is supposed to join me and where my father hands me over to him, I want it all to go smoothly. But it doesn't. Mac doesn't emerge from his seat and unaware of this, I keep on walking. When I realise that he isn't beside me, I have to walk backwards to find him. This is a manoeuvre fraught with danger and I know that I'm likely to end up flat on my back in the middle of the aisle, right in front of the poor priest.

But for once I don't fall. Mac emerges, grinning with embarrassment, joins me and we go on. The song isn't over yet. It will surely never end and I think this has already been the most fault-stricken wedding ever. And it has hardly begun yet. But I am reliably informed later, albeit by someone who wouldn't dare offend me, that it was lovely and innocent the way we looked like two children playing wedding day.

When we both promise to love, honour and cherish each other for the rest of our lives, I really mean it. I hope Mac means it too. We sign the register and leave the church. I have given explicit, implicit and strict instructions to all members of my family that I do not wish any of them to kiss me. Of course, I'd not thought to issue such instructions to Mac's family. And they are very demonstrative.

Now I know where he gets it from, only I don't know what's hit me. It seems like I'm being mobbed. And then, not to be outdone, my lot join in. What can I say or do? I just grin and bear it and think of Ireland. Here I am, married to Mac, the love of my life, and everyone is kissing me except him. The only surprise is that the priest didn't get in on the act. Well, he might as well have done. I'm sure that many of the spectators who gather to see such sport as this decided that it was too good a chance to miss.

When the usual photographs are taken we go off to the reception. The big question is, will it or won't it be there? My wedding cake, that is. Will the catering staff ever find it under the receptionist's desk if it is still there?

To my utter relief, it is there, towering over everything and looking grand. It is also going to tower over us when the time comes to cut it. My brother Tom is about to take a photograph and I hold up my hand to stop him. 'Can you see us behind the cake?' I ask in all seriousness. The guests think this is uproariously funny and I suppose it must look funny from their perspective. Anyway, we move to one side so that we can be seen.

A few hours later, when the reception is almost over – there are no speeches or any of that nonsense – we both go back to my home to change, where we sheepishly retreat to separate rooms. I have a unique going away trousseau – a pair of faithful blue denim jeans. Old, bellbottom, hipster jeans with white ducks appliquéed on the ends to be exact. I have told my family that that's what I will be wearing, but they obviously haven't believed me. My mother is mortally embarrassed. So embarrassed that she will rear up on me a year later when I go home for a visit. Mac too is wearing jeans – old raggy ones. Well, we are travelling and they seem the most ideal and comfortable for the purpose.

And so we head off. We're travelling to London, but stopping a few times on the way. Our first stop is in Nenagh, in County Tipperary which we reach in about an hour. We aren't used to the high life, we don't frequent pubs, so there is nothing to do at the hotel. We don't know what to do with ourselves. And so at 9.30 we decide to go to bed.

The room has to be vacated by noon the next morning. But my watch stops in the night and Mac doesn't have a watch, nor does he ever intend getting one. So it's one o'clock in the afternoon when we wander downstairs looking for our breakfast. Grinning all over her face, the receptionist points to the time. Mac makes things worse by explaining about the watch stopping, which seems a lame excuse, and the receptionist just keeps nodding and grinning. We pay the bill and make a run for it without breakfast or lunch.

We reach Dublin that evening, a place we're not familiar with. We drive around, find a hotel and book in. It is most embarrassing when the receptionist asks whether we want a double bed or two single beds. Mac looks at me and I feel like the proverbial Mrs. Smith or Jones. 'A double bed,' I say, bold as you like, and she now finds that the register has taken on great importance and peruses it with infinite care.

That done, we head for the dining room to have something to eat. I just want a plate of chips but Mac says they won't just serve you chips in a hotel. There are French Fries on the menu and I order them on their own and get them. But then, a moment later we realise what sort of hotel it is when we hear our car registration number being paged.

The car has been broken into. The thieves were disturbed, the swines, and little seems to be missing. Certainly the wedding presents have not been touched. It's only in the following days that we come to realise that, in fact, quite a few items have been taken. The hotel offers to allow us to bring the car right up beside the kitchens where the night porter will keep an eye on it and that will have to do for the night.

The next day we board the boat for Holyhead. I have never

been on a ship before and I feel quite certain that the car won't fit. But there are hundreds of cars on board, not to mention lorries and buses. I am amazed that the ship can float with all that weight. After all, the *Titanic* sank and there were no cars or lorries that I know of on that liner. When I mention my fears to Mac he assures me that there are no icebergs in the Irish Sea and I can't help wondering what that has got to do with anything.

Still, it's plain sailing until we arrive at Holyhead and are about to pass through customs. Here, a detective stops us. 'Where are you going?' he asks.

'To London,' Mac answers.

'What's in the car?'

'Wedding presents.'

'What type of presents?'

Mac names a few but can't remember all of them. Most of the presents had come to my house and Mac wasn't terribly interested in them. So now the detective asks me, 'What do you know about this?'

I think he's looking for an alibi for Mac, so I say, 'Well I married him.'

'I mean the list of presents,' he says, cool as you like.

'Oh those,' I say. I reel off what I can remember. I'm a bit worried that he might think me cheeky and arrest us anyway for carrying cutlery and other dangerous domestic items.

'Can I look in the back?' he now asks.

'Yes, of course,' we both say.

Mac opens the tailgate of the estate car and the detective has a quick look. He does not disturb or touch anything. Then he smiles at us, wishes us luck in our new married life and we're on our way.

We stay in a lovely motel in Wales that night. It's late when we arrive, too late for anything to eat. You may be able to get sandwiches in the bar, we are told at reception. We don't really fancy the bar, but we're starved so off we go.

As we stand there at the bar, feeling a bit sorry for ourselves, and wondering what we might do – the motel is in the middle of nowhere – we watch the barman trying to get a soda water siphon to work properly. When it does decide to work all of a sudden, the soda water squirts right on top of us. Mac comes off worse and is well drenched.

The barman is very apologetic and asks if he can do or get us anything. 'Some tea and sandwiches would be nice,' I say, cheeky as you like. The shy girl I'd been all of my life is changing. And tea and sandwiches are not a bit of bother now it seems. We can have as much as we like. And when it comes, it is just like manna from heaven.

We tour a little of north Wales the next day and it's simply beautiful. There's no shortage of mountains here – the real thing too – going thousands of feet into the sky. There is snow on Snowdonia – well, with a name like that, there should be. In the afternoon we set off on our long journey home.

Home is just two rooms and a shared bathroom. But what more could we ask for when we have love, and we're together, and we have the rest of our lives ahead of us?